Adding Neurotherapy to Your Practice

Paul G. Swingle

Adding Neurotherapy to Your Practice

Clinician's Guide to the ClinicalQ, Neurofeedback, and Braindriving

Springer

Paul G. Swingle
Swingle Clinic
Vancouver, BC, Canada

ISBN 978-3-319-15526-5 ISBN 978-3-319-15527-2 (eBook)
DOI 10.1007/978-3-319-15527-2

Library of Congress Control Number: 2015932486

Springer Cham Heidelberg New York Dordrecht London

Printed on acid-free paper

Springer International Publishing AG Switzerland is part of Springer Science+Business Media (www.springer.com)

Overview

The purpose of this book is to encourage clinicians from all licensed healthcare disciplines to consider adding basic neurotherapeutic assessment and treatment to their practices. The data are compelling, indicating that even very basic neurotherapy can markedly enhance the efficacy of most all therapeutic methods and metaphors. This book is structured to help licensed professionals learn the basic methods and principles to enable a disciplined introduction of these most efficacious therapies into their patient care modalities. The book is also focused on helping licensed professionals from falling victim to the one-size-fits-all franchise and franchise-like operations.

Neurotherapy is a data-driven methodology that is straightforward, logical, and validated by compelling research from many quarters. The procedures are based on the fact of brain plasticity, a concept that physicians and psychologists did not fully comprehend even a few short years ago. What we were taught about the brain's potential for recovery in medical and graduate schools, when I took my training, is simply wrong. Hence, many of our treatment concepts are rooted in the belief that the brain has limited capacity for functional change.

The paradigm shift implicated in the concept of neurotherapy is firmly grounded in the recent research on the plasticity of the brain. The rationale is direct and empirical: measure the functional anomalies in the brain so that one knows what symptoms the client/patient is likely to manifest. Then, treat those symptoms by normalizing the anomalous brain activity.

The procedures described in this book are quite specific and limited. Neurotherapy is a broad field with applications to many disorders. The more specialized applications are not addressed in detail, other than identifying circumstances in which one may want to refer the patient to a clinician specializing in neurotherapy.

This guide is based on a single-channel clinical grade EEG. Additional channels may be useful but are not necessary for the ClinicalQ or for the treatment that follows from the ClinicalQ analysis. Some EEG feedback systems do a very bad job of measuring the higher-frequency brain waves and others have very cumbersome software.

To proceed with introducing neurotherapy into your practice, as I am advocating in this book, you will need some basic, clinical grade equipment and the necessary basic training on the use of the equipment. My strong recommendation is that you purchase your equipment from a supplier or manufacturer that offers the basic hands-on training. Many manufacturers and suppliers have developed "turn-key" systems for the procedures presented in this book. You can contact the Biofeedback Certification International Alliance (BCIA) for a list of manufacturers and suppliers and those that offer approved hands-on training. Distance training over the net is available, but many prefer hands-on training specifically with the equipment you intend to use. Start small and work up, not the other way around. Be sure to query the supplier on the weaknesses of the system relative to the ClinicalQ requirements that are described in this book. Specifically, verify that the system measures brain wave frequencies, reliably, up to 40 Hz.

This book is divided into several sections. After a general introduction to neurotherapy in Chap. 1, Chap. 2 describes the ClinicalQ in detail. In this chapter, the conditions associated with the various brain wave patterns are presented, as well as the statistical data on the research validating the procedure. A detailed description of the diagnostic application of the ClinicalQ is emphasized in this chapter as well. Chapter 3 focuses on some of the conditions where traditional medicine and psychology have not done well following a "try this" approach to treating the labeled condition as opposed to the putative cause(s) of the client's complaints. Chapter 4 reviews the basics of neurofeedback, the "backbone" of neurotherapy. Chapter 5 focuses on methods for potentiating brain wave changes. This chapter includes the research data on identifying unconditioned stimuli for braindriving procedures, discussed in Chap. 6, as well as for procedures used for home treatment. Chapter 6 focuses on the more therapeutically aggressive braindriving techniques that use classical conditioning methods for changing brain wave activity. Chapter 7 gives a very abbreviated review of biofeedback for the peripheral systems such as thermal, muscle, and heart rate biofeedback that are very important adjunctive treatments with neurotherapy. The Appendices include the details for using the ClinicalQ in practice and evaluative questionnaires that can be used for clients. In this section as well is a review of some of the highly positively synergic interactions between pharmaceutical and neurotherapeutic approaches to treatment.

Contents

Chapter 1
Introduction

The purpose of this book is to encourage clinicians to introduce neurotherapy into their practice. Neurotherapy blends synergically with every therapeutic metaphor. Whatever your discipline, neurotherapy will markedly enhance your efficacy. As will be discussed in detail later on in this book, clinicians such as psychologists and psychiatrists, for example, will find neurotherapy markedly efficacious for treating all levels of the detrimental sequellae of exposure to severe emotional stressors.

Physicians will find that they have alternative methods for dealing with conditions such as anxiety and depression as well as facilitating greater specificity of pharmacological treatments. In the latter situation, for example, the ClinicalQ can identify the forms of ADHD that respond well to stimulants such as methylphenidate and those that do not respond well or are exacerbated by such medications. Of course, they can also incorporate neurotherapy to treat the ADHD adjunctively with medication in many instances.

This Clinician's Guide introduces clinicians to basic neurotherapy. The procedures are applicable to a broad range of patients/clients seeking treatment for a very wide array of conditions. These are basic procedures designed to augment the clinician's skill set in whatever therapeutic metaphor practiced within the jurisdictional guidelines for the professional discipline. This guide does not include more specialized areas such as full brain QEEG, z-score therapies, sLORETA, and the like. Hence, conditions such as traumatic brain injury, epilepsy, and Parkinson's require more specialized neurotherapy, although these basic procedures may be helpful in such conditions for treating adjunctive conditions such as sleep disorder, depression, and anxiety.

This guide is the sister volume to my book *Biofeedback for the Brain* (2010). The latter book is for the general public and this guide provides the technical details for clinicians. This book presents evidence from our database for the efficacy of the diagnostic procedure referred to as the "ClinicalQ." The ClinicalQ uses a limited number of EEG brain sites but provides a wealth of information about the conditions and symptoms presented by clients and patients. This procedure is not

P.G. Swingle, *Adding Neurotherapy to Your Practice*,
DOI 10.1007/978-3-319-15527-2_1

"diagnostic" in the usual understanding of that term. Rather, the ClinicalQ identifies brain functioning anomalies associated with the client's symptoms and behaviors that direct the practitioner to exact brain locations and brain wave ranges that need to be treated. It is not a labeling procedure. There is ample evidence to indicate that using the QEEG to guide treatment markedly increases the efficacy of treatment in contrast to simply relying on behavioral diagnosis (Gunkelman 2006).

Definitely NOT Business as Usual

I do not ask clients why they have come to see me. I tell them why they are seeking treatment. The level of precision of the ClinicalQ is such that, with experience, one can describe the client's condition based exclusively on the brain wave data. Clients are usually stunned by the accuracy of the description of their condition. The therapeutic value of this method is substantial. The methods have been refined over the last 20 years to the point that clients usually do not elaborate on my description of their condition.

Imagine a client who has been to many clinicians. She has told her story many times and obviously has not had much success in getting relief from her condition; otherwise, she would not be sitting in my office. She is often angry, disillusioned, depressed, and feeling hopeless. Before she can start telling her tale of woe, I say, "Do you know what I do?" I explain that I look at how the brain is functioning. I am looking for areas of inefficiency in brain activities that are, in turn, directly related to symptoms. Once identified, I correct the brain inefficiency that in turn reduces symptom intensity. I then explain that I will be looking at a few spots on the brain. She will not feel anything; it is measurement only. After I collect the brain wave data, I will do some calculations and go over the results in detail to be sure that what the brain is telling me is consistent with her personal experience. This procedure can help to commit the client to treatment. Clients are impressed by the accuracy of the diagnostic procedures and gain optimism regarding the potential efficacy of the treatment.

Many "one-size-fits-all" practitioners, many of whom are not licensed to practice any healthcare profession, treat with relaxation-focused feedback protocols. Clients may have some benefit in the short term, in terms of feeling more relaxed, but seldom achieve relief from the causes of their difficulties. As Hammond (2006b, p. 32) has pointed out, "A 'one-size-fits-all' approach that is not tailored to the individual will undoubtedly pose a greater risk of either producing an adverse reaction or of simply being ineffective." Hammond goes on to stress that anyone doing neurotherapy should be a bona fide licensed healthcare provider in the relevant jurisdiction. Hence, this book is written specifically for the licensed practitioner who wishes to add this technology to those available within her or his healthcare professional discipline.

One of my goals is to bring this effective set of therapeutic tools into the primary healthcare context so that clinicians have a broader array of options to treat many of the disorders seen on a day-to-day basis. I will describe, in precise detail, how one uses the ClinicalQ for client assessment and will show the data that validates the interpretative process. I will then proceed to describe, in detail, exactly how one does the various forms of neurotherapy to correct the conditions identified with the ClinicalQ. Neurotherapy offers the possibility to correct the problem at the source so the orientation in the treatment of some disorders like depression, for example, shifts from coping and symptom control to correcting the cause of the problem.

The term "neurotherapy" refers to a number of treatment methods that alter brain functioning. In this book we will examine many different methods for correcting brain wave anomalies. The core treatment method within this array is neurofeedback or brain wave biofeedback. All clinicians, by now, have at least a passing understanding of brain wave biofeedback. The procedure has been in use for over four decades with compelling evidence for the efficacious treatment of many disorders including epilepsy, ADHD, and depression. As we shall see, neurotherapy can be an effective alternative for the treatment of a very large array of disorders.

Neurofeedback is an operant conditioning procedure. When the brain is responding as desired, the client receives a rewarding stimulus. This can be a tone indicating positive changes in brain wave activity. The reward can also be icons moving on a computer screen so that an ADHD child, for example, is playing a video-like game with his brain. We can also create treatment preparations in which the child can keep an electric train moving with her brain. The "reward" in other words is a stimulus indicating success.

More aggressive treatment protocols include "braindriving" which is a treatment incorporating the classical conditioning processes. The classical conditioning of brain wave amplitude was demonstrated in the 1940s at McGill University in Canada by Herbert Jasper and Charles Shagass (1941). The basic preparation is to present an unconditioned stimulus contingent on brain wave activity such as amplitude. Thus, for example, when Alpha amplitude exceeds a training threshold, a flashing light is presented to the client's eyes that ceases as soon as the Alpha amplitude drops below the training threshold. Flashing light is an unconditioned stimulus for Alpha amplitude suppression. Flash a light in someone's eyes and Alpha amplitude drops. By making this process contingent on the Alpha EEG amplitude, lower amplitude can be conditioned. Much of this book will be focused on identifying the classical conditioning paradigm and the unconditioned stimuli that can be used for different brain waves at various locations.

Although clinicians may have some understanding of brain wave biofeedback, that understanding, I have found, is frequently limited. A common belief is that brain wave biofeedback is a good, but costly, method to help patients relax. More efficient than meditation, it nonetheless has a limited benefit of a temporary change in brain wave activity, similar to drowsiness that helps clients find a relaxing state. Inherent in this conception is that brain wave biofeedback does not affect permanent change in brain wave functioning. Thus, clinicians with this misconception of brain wave biofeedback are likely to dismiss neurotherapy as simply another form of relaxation.

Neurotherapy treats conditions that have been considered untreatable. These methods can provide more effective ways for treating many of the depression and anxiety disorders than conventional psychology and medicine have offered to date. But neurotherapy does not replace these traditional methods; rather, it offers opportunities for synergy among the treatment methods.

Neurotherapeutic treatment starts with an assessment of brain wave activity. We have an understanding of what that brain wave activity should look like under normal circumstances. Departures from those normative values are indicative of some level of inefficiency in brain functioning. These inefficiencies in brain functioning in turn are associated with symptoms. By interpreting these departures from normative values, the clinician can identify the symptoms that brought the patient to seek treatment. It is very different from the usual procedure of the client describing the problems to the clinician. After verifying that the symptoms suggested by the brain wave anomalies are those for which the client seeks treatment, the clinician proceeds to outline, to the patient, the exact nature of the treatments designed to normalize the brain wave activity that in turn leads to symptom improvement.

An initial decision that must be taken at the outset is whether or not the patient needs to have a full head electroencephalography (all 19 sites, called a FullQ, or full map) or if the limited ClinicalQ will be adequate. Conditions of traumatic brain injury, including head trauma and stroke, certainly would require the FullQ. Similarly, conditions such as seizure disorders and psychoses likewise should be assessed with the FullQ. Conditions more commonly seen, including the anxiety disorders, the various forms of depression, attention problems in children, panic disorders, irritable and inflammatory bowel disorders, sleep quality issues, addictions, fibromyalgia, chronic fatigue, and the sequellae of emotional trauma, all would be appropriate to assess with the ClinicalQ.

Brain Wave Biofeedback

Brain wave biofeedback, also called neurofeedback, is based on a simple premise that clients can alter a brain wave activity if they receive immediate feedback on brain wave state changes. We have known since the mid-1960s that rodents can be taught to change their heart rate and blood pressure (Dicara and Miller 1969). And from around that same time, we have known that cats can be taught to change their brain wave activity (Sterman 2000). Evidence that such changes are stable over time, an indicator of brain plasticity (LeDoux 2002), was reported some years later (Lubar 1991).

If clients can be taught to change their brain wave activity, and such changes are stable over time, then symptoms associated with an abnormal brain wave activity should be treatable by normalizing brain waves. The clinical procedures are remarkably logical and straightforward: measure the brain wave activity; find the anomalies; ask the patient if the symptoms associated with the identified anomalies are present; and if the client admits to the symptoms, then help the client learn to correct the anomalies with brainwave biofeedback. When the anomalies are corrected (brain wave activity within normative ranges), the patient should report symptom elimination or improvement.

We will be looking at a limited number of brain wave ranges for diagnostic purposes. The important ranges are Delta (2 cycles per second, Hz), Alpha (8–12 Hz), Theta (3–7 Hz), Beta (16–25 Hz), and high Beta/Gamma (28–40 Hz). Some other more limited ranges will be considered as well. As will become obvious, the significance of each of these brain wave ranges depends on the brain location. For example, elevated Theta in the front part of the brain may be associated with poor cognitive processing, whereas similar amplitude of Theta in the back of the brain may be associated with feelings of calm and well-being. Similarly, too much Alpha in the right frontal cortex may be associated with defiance in a child, whereas similar amplitude in the left may be associated with depressed mood state.

Once the problematic areas are determined, the practitioner selects the appropriate brain wave ranges that are to be treated and sets the treatment parameters so the patient receives feedback for the desired brain wave changes in real time. For example, a client with an alcohol problem who has a brain wave deficiency in the back of the brain would have the electrode placed over the occipital region. In such cases the problem is often a deficiency of Theta amplitude (brain waves between 3 and 7 Hz) or an excess of Beta amplitude (brain waves between 16 and 25 Hz), so the practitioner would set the training parameters to give a tone feedback whenever the amplitude of Theta is increasing and/or the amplitude of Beta is decreasing. Patients generally do this kind of brain wave biofeedback with eyes closed.

Stimulated EEG (Braindriving)

All stimulation changes brain waves. Stimulation, such as sound, can have a specific effect on brain waves, and this specificity can be used systematically to condition brain activity. One of the most important developments in neurotherapeutic treatment procedures, stimulated EEG procedures, called braindriving, can rapidly modify brain wave activity. These procedures are often used for emergencies to calm distressed clients and are particularly effective with autistic spectrum disordered clients. In addition, braindriving is used in remediation protocols, in which brain stimulation is occurring simultaneously with a task such as reading or writing.

The basic principle of braindriving is that stimulation is contingent on brain wave activity, in contrast to a static procedure of stimulation independent of brain wave activity. For example, one can listen to music, a static situation, and measure changes in EEG activity associated with the stimulation. In a braindriving preparation, the stimulating music would be presented only when a specific brain wave condition prevailed. The music would shut off if the specific brain wave condition were not present.

For example, severely distraught clients often need immediate relief. These clients may be in states of anxiety, panic, fatigue, despair, or physical unease. A psychologist might attempt to provide relief by guiding the client in a relaxation exercise or by administering a quieting procedure such as hypnosis, craniosacral therapy, bilateral stimulation, experiential therapy, microamperage stimulation of the head or of acupuncture points, or one of the several energy psychology procedures. A physician might also consider medicating the patient. Generally, these procedures are used to quiet the patient, after which the patient is engaged in some therapeutic procedures to correct the cause of the distress.

Braindriving offers an effective method for bringing immediate relief in such situations, as exemplified in the following case of a client who was experiencing severe anxiety and deep depression. She reported that she was crying "continuously," could not sleep, and was having panic episodes. The condition had come on suddenly and she was frightened and considered going to an emergency room at a psychiatric hospital. She reported a history of depression and always felt that she was an anxious person.

When using braindriving in this acute context, it is critical that the client understands that the procedure is designed to give significant but temporary relief and that they must commit to engaging in therapy to deal with the neurological and psychological causes of distress. When dealing with urgent situations of clients in severe distress, the usual ClinicalQ brain wave evaluation is abbreviated. The clinician reads the data and moves directly to the treatment without providing assessment information to the client. Clients in states of severe distress are not in a position to benefit from a detailed explanation of their brain wave patterns, and eliminating it provides more time for the emergency treatment. The brain wave data are explained in detail to the client at the next session, after the client has regained some calm and composure. Acute decompensation is routinely associated with a frontal lobe imbalance and a deficiency in the slow brain wave frequencies and/or an excess of fast-frequency amplitude in the back of the brain.

After verifying that these brain wave conditions prevail, the clinician moves directly to administering the emergency treatment to calm the client. In the present case, the frontal Alpha was found to be imbalanced with the left, having 26.9 % greater Alpha amplitude relative to the right, and the Theta/Beta ratio at location O1 in the occipital region was 0.66. As will be discussed in detail later in this book, these values are considerably outside the clinical normative ranges. The emergency braindriving combined the treatment of both the frontal lobes and the occipital region. At the end of the 40-min treatment, the frontal lobes were balanced and the ratio in the back of the brain had more than doubled. Even though still deficient in the Theta/Beta ratio at the back, the client reported considerable relief from her distress and was able to resume her day-to-day activities while she proceeded with psychological treatment. She was scheduled for a return visit in 2 days at which time her data would be reviewed, and a brief version of the emergency treatment administered to help sustain the improved calm.

At the core of my approach to neurotherapy is the ClinicalQ. Simply stated, the ClinicalQ is a very efficient intake assessment methodology. It provides rapid diagnostic data that permits remarkably accurate descriptions of the client's complaints without asking the client to explain anything. Of critical importance to any clinician treating disorders of the central and autonomic nervous systems, the rapport with the client/patient is profoundly strengthened with the use and interpretation of the ClinicalQ during the intake session.

The ClinicalQ is rapid, requiring only 6½ min of recording time when using a single EEG channel and considerably less time when using multiple channels. It is data driven and logical and offers not only diagnostic insights but also serves as a guide to precise treatment and a method to evaluate patient progress as treatment proceeds. We turn now to a detailed discussion of the ClinicalQ and the research supporting the interpretations of the data obtained from this efficient assessment procedure.

Chapter 2
The ClinicalQ

Clinical Versus Normative Databases

For clinicians, the most accurate databases are clearly clinical. Normative databases are far less accurate. The fundamental organizing concept of the normative database for the clinical practitioner is, simply stated, wrong.

The organizing concept for normative databases is that one can identify a group of individuals who are symptom free and therefore have "normal" functioning neurology. This group of symptom free individuals then serves as the comparative database to identify those who are statistically discriminant. The statistical departures from the normative database define the anomalous neurological condition that is associated either causatively or exacerbatitively with the client's clinical condition. This concept is wrong.

The reason that normative database treatment recommendations are so often incorrect is because the fundamental premise is wrong. Symptom free individuals may well have predispositions to conditions that have not manifested. The data are quite clear and we have definitive evidence for this that spans decades.

Let us simply take the example of heritability data for schizophrenia. As the data in Table 2.1 indicate, if one monozygotic twin has been diagnosed with schizophrenia the probability that the second identical twin will have schizophrenia is about 50 %. But, the interesting statistic is that 50 % will not! Where do we find the 50 % without manifested schizophrenia, but obviously with the same genetic load? In the normative databases! So clearly the organizing concept for normative databases, at least for clinicians, is incorrect. Normative databases so constituted ignore basic psychopathology and basic biology. Every person has predispositions. Predispositions to anxiety, depression, emotional volatility, and the like. However, many of these predispositions are not manifest at any particular time. In general, clinicians understand that one needs an experiential trigger to "turn-the-key" to manifest a neurological predisposition.

P.G. Swingle, *Adding Neurotherapy to Your Practice*,
DOI 10.1007/978-3-319-15527-2_2

Table 2.1 Heritability statistics on schizophrenia

Genetic predispositions	
Monozygotic twins	30–50 %
Dizygotic twins	15 %
Siblings	15 %
General population	1 %

Adopted-biological relatives with Schizophrenia	
Adoptee with Schizophrenia	13 %
Adoptee without Schizophrenia	2 %

Source: Gottesman (1991) *Schizophrenia Genesis: The Origin of Madness*. New York: Freeman.

These logic considerations are well known and surprisingly, at least to me, ignored by non-clinicians that develop the normative databases. If in the normative database one has subjects with non-manifested predispositions, then statistically one can expect very poor discrimination.

Conditional Probability Models

There are many conditional probability models associated with the concepts of differential susceptibility. In mathematical game theory, the probability of future actions is predicated on present state. In chess, the probability of Queen move is markedly different if Queen Pawn has advanced. This is considered a state conditional probability.

In optimal performance contexts, conditional probability theories consider both vulnerability as well as resilience markers. The markers can be direct, or primary, such as the genetic serotonergic system inefficiency affecting stress tolerance. The concept of "preparation for duty" for military and police personnel is premised on reducing vulnerability to work stress (e.g., combat) by increasing the neurological basis for stress tolerance.

Secondary markers may be introversion that reduces probability of development of social relationships that in turn is negatively synergic with the primary marker. Hence, in the latter case the individual who has experienced severe stress may be more vulnerable to negative posttraumatic sequellae if the secondary marker impeded the development of a social support network.

Obviously, in the clinical context, individuals who present themselves for treatment have a manifested susceptibility factor. Individuals who do not present for treatment may have the same neurological predisposition but has not manifested. Hence, the latter individual is a candidate for normative database whereas his cohort with the identical, but manifested, predisposition is in my office and hence in the clinical database. Also, obvious, the normative database is going to be statistically blind to many neurological conditions that are predispositions.

Where normative databases have strength are determinant neurological abnormalities such as those associated with epilepsy, autism, structural damage, and progressive neurological deterioration. Conditions associated with primary genetic (e.g., dopamine/serotonin), secondary endophenotypic (e.g., autonomic reactivity) and phenotypic (e.g., sensory processing), and tertiary endomorphic (e.g., body mass) are likely to be under the statistical discrimination thresholds. However, most importantly, the normative databases just simply miss neurological relationships found in brainwave activity for conditions that bring clients into the clinician's office.

The ClinicalQ is a clinical database. The database contains 1,508 clinical clients. The organizing logic is that clients who report a condition (e.g., depression) have a neurological representation of that condition. Based on the diathesis vulnerability model, the condition reported by the client is one that is associated with a neurological predisposition that has manifested. A normative database is likely to miss this entirely since this clinical client, before becoming depressed, had the same neurological predisposition but would be considered "normal" (i.e., symptom free) and eligible for the normative database.

The important concepts of the vulnerability or conditional probability models for the clinician include conditional vulnerability (cf., Ingram and Luxton 2005), diathesis (Sigelman and Rider 2009; Belsky and Pluess 2009) and that although neurological predispositions are stable across the lifespan, they are not unchangeable (Lipton 2006; Oatley et al. 2006).

Although the theoretical concepts associated with predispositions and vulnerabilities are of interest, for the purposes of this guide, the critical issues are that predispositions are just that, predispositions. It is also important that predisposition does not mean inevitable. People can have a multitude of predispositions but may be fortunate enough to never have them triggered and therefore be even more fortunate to never need our services.

Finally, expressivity of the predisposition in neurology is analogous to severity of a condition in clinical medicine. The severity of the EEG condition is not directly associated with the severity of the symptom. In general, the more severe the EEG condition, the more pronounced the symptomatology in terms of several parameters including chronicity, intensity, treatment resistance, and qualitative manifestation. However, many variations occur so that clinically one uses the ClinicalQ to identify clinical conditions that should be probed/explored with the client. The qualitative features of the symptoms may well be poorly correlated with the magnitude of the ClinicalQ markers. This is especially true of ClinicalQ markers associated with experiential factors as compared to genetic predispositions.

The ClinicalQ

Introduction

To illustrate the superiority of clinical norms, consider the following comparison with a normative database (Figs. 2.1, 2.2, and 2.3). Both the ClinicalQ and the 19-point full EEG were obtained simultaneously. The normative report was generated by one of the best known services whereas the ClinicalQ was generated

NAME: M 21 **DATE:** 10/27/04

Please list the symptoms for which you are seeking treatment. Indicate the severity of the symptoms according to the following scale.

1 = A minor problem.
2 = Distressing, but I can usually ignore the problem.
3 = Serious and occasionally interferes with social or work activities.
4 = Very serious and often interferes with social or work activities.
5 = Completely interferes with work and social activities.

For example, if you experience sleep disturbances that occasionally leave you too fatigues to participate in social functions, but has never prevented you from working, your listing might be as follows:

Problem/Symptom	**Severity**
"Problem with falling into sleep and I wake often and find it difficult to get back to sleep."	3

Problem/Symptom	**Severity**
1. Problem Falling asleep, and Staying asleep	4
2. I get angry easily	4
3. I have trouble concentrating or Staying focused	4.

Fig. 2.1 Client's (M21) self-reported conditions

II. Conclusion:

The background alpha is seen at 9-10 Hz with eyes closed, with frontal theta seen maximally at the midline anteriorly overlying the cingulate, and with persistent EMG artifact fronto-temporally and posteriorly, as described. There is less beta power than expected. The frontal midline slower content is described in perseverative disturbances such as OCD/ODD and the over-focus associated with generalized anxiety disorder. The theta/beta ratio was increased significantly, as is commonly seen in AD/HD at the vertex. There is left mu noted, which is a normal neurological variant, though it is also reported disproportionately in those with mirror neuron disturbances. There is a slight increase in the relative slower content left temporally, suggesting a disturbance in areas involved in language comprehension and verbal memory.

III. Recommendation for therapy:

Based on these findings, the SMR training should be considered for stabilization and calming, and to help re-tune the alpha frequencies. The left temporal training may be added to address any language comprehension or verbal memory issues**. The frontal midline slower suppression with beta training may be used for stimulation, as well as to counter-act any under-activation noted due to the SMR type training. The faster beta suppression band is intended to catch the EMG activity noted during the recording.

The specific frequencies, montages, and the sequencing of sessions will likely require modification based on client response. Suggestions may be implemented differently depending on instrumentation used. All decisions regarding implementation of these suggestions are the responsibility of the practitioner. *I recognize the need for on-going consultation and welcome discussion concerning clinical progress of individual patients, or related questions and suggestions.*

	Active	Reference	train	inhibit
1	Cz	Linked ears	(12-15)	(5-11) + (22-30)
2	T5 **	Cz	(13-16)	(5-11) + (22-30)
3	Fz	Linked ears	(15-18)	(5-11) + (22-30)

** The T5 is for language comprehension, as well as verbal memory.

Fig. 2.2 Client M21. Full 19-site QEEG report from independent service using normative database

CZ	VALUES
EO Alpha	7.1
EC Alpha	10.2
% Change EO to EC Alpha	43.7
EO Alpha Recovery %	8.3
EO Theta/Beta	2.94
UT Theta/Beta	3.11
% Change T/B EO to T/B UT	5.8
Total Amplitude	33.6
Alpha Peak Frequency EC	9.3
Alpha Peak Frequency EO	9.1
Theta/SMR EC	2.45

O1	VALUES
Alpha EO	9.2
Alpha EC	14.3
% Change in Alpha EO to EC	53.7
EO Alpha Recovery %	15.3
Theta/Beta EO	2.21
Theta/Beta EC	1.26
% Change T/B EO to T/B EC	75.4
Alpha Peak Frequency EO	9.6

F3 & F4 (ALL EC)	VALUES		% Difference
	F3	F4	F3-F4
Alpha Amplitude	8.9	12.3	38.2
Beta Amplitude	6.8	8.4	23.5
Theta Amplitude	22.9	21.4	7.0
Theta/Beta	3.37	2.55	32.2

FZ (ALL EC)	VALUES
Delta (2 Hz)	17.2
HiBeta/Beta	0.48
Sum HiBeta + Beta	14.2
LoAlpha/HiAlpha	1.75
Alpha Peak Frequency	9.4

Fig. 2.3 ClinicalQ for client M21

immediately while the client was still hooked up. Many manufacturers of EEG platforms have software available for generating the ClinicalQ data and probes; however, following the outline in the Appendix one can generate the ClinicalQ data and summary with any EEG platform with the aid of a desktop hand calculator.

It is quite apparent that the ClinicalQ was far more accurate for this client. He reported sleep problems consistent with the low Theta/Beta ratio under eyes-closed conditions at location O1. The marked imbalance in Alpha, frontally, with Alpha being considerably higher in amplitude in the right relative to the left is the marker for emotional volatility. As this client reports: "I get angry easily." The client's complaints of problems with focus and attention are reflected in the elevated Theta/Beta ratios at location Cz, F3, and F4 as well as the elevated Delta and slow Alpha as measured at Fz.

We also see another marker that is not reported by the client. Beta is considerably greater in amplitude in the right relative to the left frontal cortex. This is a marker for depression. When probed about this, the client admitted to feeling "low" much more intensely and frequently then he believed was the case with his friends.

The ClinicalQ shows precisely where to treat these conditions and what to treat: Standard Theta/Beta training at locations Cz, and if necessary later at F3 and F4. Increasing the Theta/Beta ratio at O1, eyes closed, for the sleep problems. Speed up the Alpha peak frequency (or decrease the amplitude of low Alpha) and finally balance the frontal regions, F3 and F4, in the Alpha and Beta ranges. Rule of thumb—treat sleep problems first as restored sleep quality is likely to result in other improvements in brain functioning. There are many other general guidelines for how to approach developing a treatment strategy for the clients that will be discussed more specifically later in this book.

It is also apparent that the QEEG report not only did not identify the client's complaints but the treatment strategy recommended is largely irrelevant to the client's problems. The possible exception is the recommended 12–15 Hz training at Cz. However, neurofeedback at almost any location is usually associated with client reports of improvement early in treatment.

So, it is obvious that the ClinicalQ is *not* a poor practitioner's substitution for the full 19-site QEEG. Many mini-Q systems are being marketed on exactly that basis. The purpose of using the ClinicalQ is to make neurotherapy much more efficient; because, again, the ClinicalQ is more accurate for clinical practice than the normative databases.

The intake procedure with the ClinicalQ is the first therapy session. Clients are strongly relieved that their complaints are understood, that there are identifiable neurological causes/corollaries of their condition, and there is a precise "game plan" for treatment. The average length of treatment at the Swingle Clinic for most conditions is about 23 sessions, and for simple problems like Common ADD (CADD) it is closer to 15, which is far below industry standards (Swingle 2002). This efficiency is based on many aspects and modalities of treatment such as the use of braindriving techniques and the home treatment procedures described in later chapters. However, a major contributor to that efficiency is the ClinicalQ at the initial visit.

When clients present for treatment, they generally expect to have to spend at least one, perhaps several, sessions telling their tales of woe and submitting to various forms of assessment. Imagine their pleasant surprise when they experience something so radically different, yet so logically sound, as letting the brain diagnose their problem. As I will detail later in this chapter, one can literally tell the client why he or she came to your office without any report from them and with less than 10 min of EEG recording.

Again, the reason for the unique accuracy and efficiency of the ClinicalQ is because this assessment is based on clinical norms. For all of the reasons discussed above, for intake of clinical clients, normative databases are simply too imprecise.

After telling clients why they are sitting across from you, you can point out how you knew what the problems were and exactly what areas of brain functioning are going to be modified to correct those problems. Treatment can start immediately, certainly in terms of home treatments, and often with brief neurotherapy at the very same first visit. Quite a departure from their experience with other healthcare providers. In addition, the client knows that brainwave assessment has efficacy because you have accurately and completely described the symptoms relying only on the ClinicalQ.

A number of clinicians have shown that there are identifiable EEG patterns associated with a variety of physical and psychological disorders. Deficient Alpha power in schizophrenics has consistently been reported, for example, and EEG slowing is a good indicator of degree of cognitive impairment (Hughes and John 1999). Similarly, specific EEG patterns have been shown to be associated with various forms of ADD (Thompson and Thompson 2006; Swingle 2010), learning disabilities (Thornton 2006), and physical disorders (Hammond 2006a). Thus, like neurofeedback, diagnostic use of the EEG has a research base extending over many years.

The database for the ClinicalQ diagnostic procedures is very large in comparison to some of the previous studies. With over 1,500 patients, the sample size for the ClinicalQ database exceeds even some of the QEEG databases. Further, the ClinicalQ procedure avoids diagnostic labels and categorizing but focuses rather on the behavioral manifestations of the inefficiencies found in brain activity.

When clients present for treatment, the vast majority do not really care if their brainwave architecture departs from normative values. Moreover, sometimes the problem resides in brainwave activity that is not outside normative ranges as determined by the databases. For the reasons discussed above, normative ranges may be statistically insensitive to discriminative patters associated with symptoms. Hence, reliance on normative databases can result in missing areas of opportunity for neurotherapy.

Clients want their problems resolved regardless of normative EEG values. Many clients have endured various healthcare providers' efforts to deal with their problems, often with repetitive intake evaluations that are time- and money consuming. Imagine how they might feel about your potential for helping them if you tell them more about their problems within 30 min than others have been able to tell them after many sessions and/or assessment procedures.

Dramatic instances of clients being shocked by this highly efficient intake procedure occur when the ClinicalQ record shows the "trauma signature." The details associated with the trauma signature will be described in detail later in this chapter, but basically it is a marked absence of Alpha amplitude under eyes-closed conditions. Imagine the client's surprise when, after a few minutes of recording, the practitioner asks if they have a history of emotional trauma. The accuracy rate associated with the trauma signature is good. In the words of one physician who recently introduced the ClinicalQ into his practice, the procedure vastly expands the therapeutic options because of a profoundly expanded understanding of the patient, which the patient recognizes.

Words from a Mom on the ClinicalQ Assessment

Susan Olding
From her book "*Pathologies*" Freehand Press

Desperate, determined, undeterred by cost or lack of insurance coverage, undismayed by the doubts of conventional physicians, undaunted by the practitioner's Dickensian-sounding name, I switched off my cell phone at the threshold of Dr. Swingle's office and carried my daughter across…

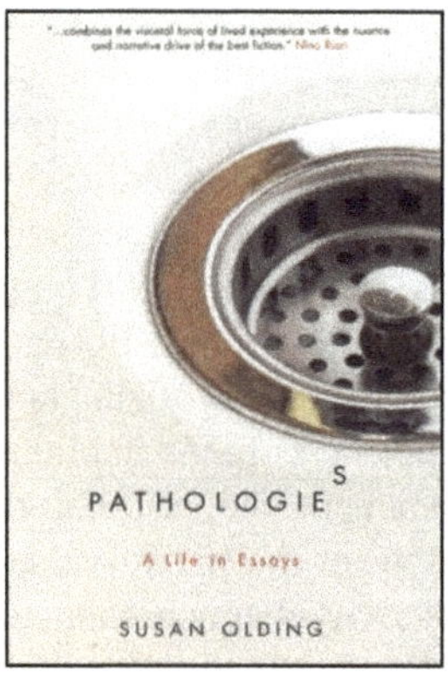

I had brought a medical and developmental history—the long litany of concerns that had brought us to his door—but Dr. Swingle waved the papers aside without even looking at them. Instead, he ushered Maia toward a computer screen on the other side of the room and told her to put her feet on the stool below. Then he fixed a couple of delicate wires to her ears…

Then Dr. Swingle sent Maia to the "treasure chest" in the waiting room. He stared at the printout in his hand. "Here," he said, and he pointed to an outline of the brain, "These numbers imply trauma." He shrugged, palms up, waiting for my response. I nodded. "And here," he continued, "too much theta. This is the hyperactivity people associate with ADHD. But it's minor. In the ballpark I play in, she barely makes the field." There was more: extreme stubbornness, a tendency to perseverate, lapses of short-term memory, attachment disorder, inability to read social cues, emotional reactivity, tantrums, explosions. One by one he read the ratios, divining[1] my daughter's character—more quickly, more accurately than any professional I'd yet encountered.

The ClinicalQ does not replace the full QEEG. We often do a full QEEG on clients after 10 or so sessions. We do so to assess therapeutic progress but also to provide further interpretative opportunities offered by 19 sites of data. For example, many clients have difficulties that may be more efficiently addressed by treating problems with coherence in the brain. Coherence refers to the degree of interaction, or communication, between brain sites. Hyper-coherence is when the brain sites are not functioning in an efficient interdependent fashion, but rather have too much "cross-talk." This condition is often found with brain injury, after which clients experience stereotypical, perseverative, and inflexible behavior and cognitive processing. Hypo-coherence, poor inter-site interaction, is associated with diminished cognitive efficiency. To assess coherence in the brain, a full QEEG is required.

However, even if I start with a full QEEG, I always provide the client with immediate feedback based on the data analyses of the ClinicalQ. I do so, as stressed above, for purely therapeutic reasons. Even though clients may have to wait for the QEEG assessment, as they do for virtually all other medical and psychological tests, they get immediate feedback regarding their major complaints on the spot with all of the benefits discussed above. Further, more than 80 % of our clients never need the full QEEG because of the efficiency of the ClinicalQ.

The ClinicalQ Procedure

As with any assessment, it is very important to follow the procedure precisely. It is critical to the interpretative probes that the brainwave ranges and EEG sites are as specified in this guide. Unfortunately, some EEG systems have fixed ranges that are slightly different from these and are very difficult to modify. Any deviation from the specified brainwave ranges and EEG sites reduces the efficacy of the procedure.

The length of each measurement epoch is usually 15 s, but this can be modified if necessary. For example, if assessing a child who cannot stay still, one can shorten the measurement epoch and select those with minimal movement.

All of the measurements are in microvolt amplitude, and the ratios are robust across different systems. The summated values, such as Total Amplitude (TA) (i.e., sum of three brainwave bands as described below), may vary from system to system,

---

[1] Although I am flattered by the divine/prophetic reference, I believe that Susan meant the more secular meaning: Divination can be seen as a systematic method with which to organize what appear to be disjointed, random facets of existence such that they provide insight into a problem at hand.

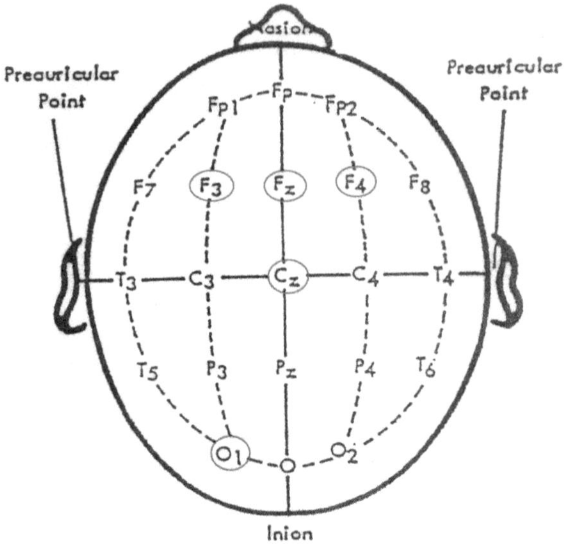

Fig. 2.4 10–20 international EEG site location system. The five-point ClinicalQ locations are noted in red (Colour figure online)

and certainly among the different filtering options, so the clinician may find it necessary to find equivalent power ranges.

The essential brainwave ranges to measure are Delta (2 Hz), Theta (3–7 HZ), Alpha (8–12 Hz), Sensory Motor Rhythm (SMR) (13–15 Hz), Beta (16–25 Hz), HiBeta-Gamma (28–40 Hz), Lo-Alpha (8–9 Hz), and Hi-Alpha (11–12 Hz). All these ranges need not be measured at all sites. The ClinicalQ only requires three bands at any particular site. The sites are Cz, O1, F3, F4, and Fz, using the 10–20 international system, as shown in Fig. 2.4.

To illustrate the bottom-up assessment procedure, as described by Susan Olding in the above excerpt from her book, consider the following data from an actual client. As emphasized by Susan Olding when I assessed her child, I know nothing about this child other than he is 14 years old and not at all happy about having been dragged into my office by his mother. Let's call him Mitch, not his actual name, of course.

As noted in the schematic shown in Fig. 2.4, these numbers are from five brain locations: the top of the head (Cz), the back of the head (O1), and the left (F3) and the right (F4) and the middle (Fz) of the front of the head. The measurement requires just over 6 min of recording time and the tasks are simple (open and close the eyes and read something out loud).

In our workshops teaching other clinicians to use the clinical QEEG procedure, we always emphasize that neurotherapy is not a standalone procedure. In short, I tell clinicians "Don't leave your clinical hat at the door when you do neurotherapy." During the first session with this child, for example, all I had to do was look at him to know that he was experiencing difficulties. He was sullen and would not make eye contact with me. He slouched in the chair, looking as disinterested as he could, looking out of the window and yawning. His mother was anxious to tell me all about his difficulties.

It is very important in these circumstances not to validate the child's expectations. What this child was expecting was for his mother to go through her tale of woe telling me all of the difficulties that the child has had and all of the difficulties she and/or the family has had with regard to the behavior of this child. As described in Susan Olding's account of her experience with the ClinicalQ, I did not permit the mother to proceed with her account describing the child's behavior; rather, I addressed the child directly.

Often with young children, if you address the issue of sports, you can start to develop some sort of relationship. Unfortunately, in our present digital culture this is becoming less likely as many children, particularly those we see for treatment, are addicted to the internet and have little interest in sports. In this case, I asked the child what sports he played and I was very fortunate that he mentioned soccer. This provided me with my first possible inroad to being able to get this child to acknowledge his difficulties and address the problems. I pointed out that the team that had won the World Cup in soccer in the year 2006 (soccer team from Milan, Italy), every player on the team had done neurotherapy—the same therapy with which he is likely to be involved. I went on to describe some of the other uses of neurofeedback including the local hockey team and the Olympic athletes who were going to participate in the Winter Olympics in Vancouver, Canada. At this point, the child was attentive to me but still rather solemn and not responding with anything but grunts and head nods.

After this brief introduction, I brought the child over to the area where we do the brain assessment and simply told him that he would feel nothing, that this was measurement only, and that it would not take much time. I also pointed out that I would be asking him to open and close his eyes at various times and to read something out loud. I also pointed out that the measurement is movement-sensitive and to try to be as still as possible during the measurement procedure.

The raw data shown in Fig. 2.5 are the result of that assessment. The raw data consists of 99 numbers, and these 99 numbers are reduced to 30 summary markers that are shown in Fig. 2.6.

We will be reviewing a great many data recordings of children with all manner of neurological issues that adversely affect their ability to pay attention and to learn. We will also be examining a great many records of children whose problems are emotional and behavioral in nature and not primarily the result of neurological problems. For the present purposes, the basic data recording will be reviewed to illustrate how profoundly accurate and sensible the ClinicalQ EEG method is, relative to the ubiquitous top-down methods. The actual data calculations are also presented so the reader can appreciate how straightforward and uncomplicated the procedure is for obtaining the ClinicalQ. The specific items that facilitated the precision of diagnosis will be identified but just the essentials that guided the evaluation of this child's presenting complaints. These essential indicators are circled in red to set them apart from the other summary statistics.

As we proceed through the book looking at a number of different cases, the significance of all of these summary numbers will become apparent. For the present purposes, we want to focus only on those that have been highlighted, to demonstrate

Cz — MALE 13 YO

Average Amplitudes:	THETA	ALPHA	BETA
Trial #	Filter 1 uV	Filter 2 uV	Filter 3 uV
1	21.1	12.8	8.0
2	19.4	15.0	6.3
3	29.0	19.5	8.6
4	22.1	14.8	7.4
5	18.3	13.0	8.5
6	23.5	12.1	7.6
7	20.4	12.5	8.0
8	19.1	12.1	8.9
9	20.4	13.2	8.2
10	19.9	15.8	7.2
Session Avg.	21.3	14.1	7.9

O1

Average Amplitudes:	THETA	ALPHA	BETA	
Trial #	Filter 1 uV	Filter 2 uV	Filter 3 uV	
1	17.8	16.2	7.5	
2	16.0	14.7	7.7	
3	28.0	34.2	10.1	
4	19.8	17.7	7.4	
5	22.9	15.1	7.1	F4
6	22.0	15.8	7.8	F4
7	22.6	17.1	7.7	F4
8	22.7	17.2	7.0	F3
9	17.6	12.7	7.0	F3
10	21.3	17.1	7.2	F3
Session Avg.	21.1	17.8	7.6	

Fz

Average Amplitudes:	DELTA	28-40Hz	BETA
Trial #	Filter 1 uV	Filter 2 uV	Filter 3 uV
1	10.3	4.1	6.1
2	6.8	4.0	6.7
3	9.7	4.3	6.5
4	8.2	3.8	6.0
5	7.0	4.4	6.6
6	14.2 LOW ALPHA	4.8 HIGH ALPHA	18.1 THETA
7	13.3	5.3	21.9
8	13.6	6.8	25.9
9	12.2	7.3	23.8
10	15.9	5.6	20.6
Session Avg.	11.1	5.0	14.2

Fig. 2.5 Raw data from ClinicalQ recording of a 14-year-old male

the remarkable efficiency of allowing the brain to tell us what the problems are, and where to go to fix them. The first indicators are at location Cz, directly on top of the head. The first number, 2.70, is the ratio of the amplitude of Theta (brainwaves from 3 to 7 cycles per second) divided by the amplitude of Beta (brainwaves from 16 to 25 cycles per second). The Theta/Beta ratio is extremely important in that it gives us an indication of the level of arousal of specific areas of the brain. We have databases for normative values for the normal functioning brain. The Theta/Beta ratio at that location for a child of about 14 years of age should be below about 2.20. Mitch's ratio is 2.70. What this tells us is that this child has some difficulty associated with focus. When that area of the brain is hypoactive as indicated by elevated Theta/Beta

CZ	VALUES
EO Alpha	15.0
EC Alpha	19.5
% Change EO to EC Alpha	30.0
EO Alpha Recovery %	-1.3
EO Theta/Beta	2.70
UT Theta/Beta	3.09
% Change T/B EO to T/B UT	14.4

O1	VALUES
Alpha EO	14.7
Alpha EC	34.2
% Change in Alpha EO to EC	132.6
EO Alpha Recovery %	20.4
Theta/Beta EO	2.08
Theta/Beta EC	2.77
% Change T/B EO to T/B EC	33.2

F3 & F4 (ALL EC)	VALUES		% Difference
	F3	F4	F3-F4
Beta Amplitude	7.0	7.7	10.0
Alpha Amplitude	17.1	15.8	8.2
Theta Amplitude	21.3	22.6	6.1
Theta/Beta Ratio	3.04	2.94	3.4

FZ (ALL EC)	VALUES
Delta (2 Hz)	8.2
HiBeta/Beta	0.63
Sum HiBeta + Beta	10.6
LoAlpha/HiAlpha	2.43

Fig. 2.6 Summary statistics for the ClinicalQ shown in Fig. 2.5. Areas of diagnostic importance highlighted in red (Colour figure online)

ratio, there is too much slow activity and/or too little fast activity. This indicates that Mitch is facing a challenge in terms of focus, concentration, attention, and staying on target. If that ratio was considerably greater, up in the range of four or so, we would likely be probing to determine if Mitch is hyperactive. However, in the present case it is more likely that Mitch's ADHD is of the inattentive variety.

What is most critical in this particular profile is the second number on that line, which is 3.09. This is the Theta/Beta ratio that was obtained when the child was under cognitive challenge. This was done during the time that he was asked to read aloud. Notice that the number increased from 2.70 to 3.09.

This is a particularly pernicious form of ADHD. When under cognitive challenge such as reading, the brain should be producing less slow frequency (i.e., lower amplitude or strength) associated with hypoactivity and/or greater fast activity associated with focus and attention. When it goes the opposite way (the ratio of the amplitude of slow frequency vs. high frequency gets larger), then this is a condition in which the harder the child tries, the worse the situation gets. We tend to find this condition mostly in males. The curious feature of this form of ADHD is that in some clients there are conditions in which the brain looks absolutely fine. The only time one sees the anomalous brainwave activity is when the child is being cognitively challenged. Thus, measuring brainwave activity when the child is simply sitting and not engaged does not reveal the condition that is causing the problems. Only when the child is asked to read aloud, or to count, do we see the elevated slow frequency amplitude.

The person who discovered this form of ADD is Professor George Fitzsimmons of the University of Alberta. The number of children who show the pattern just described (only see ADHD EEG profiles when being cognitively challenged) is not large. In most cases, one also sees neurological ADHD patterns even when the child is at rest. The important feature of this condition, however, is that cognitive challenge intensifies the condition. The usual result of this is that the harder the child tries, the worse the situation becomes. When trying to concentrate, the brain is showing greater amplitude of a brainwave that is associated with daydreaming and early stages of sleep. The tragic result is that children like this are highly at risk for simply giving up. They make determined efforts to keep up, and despite these efforts, they fall behind. These kids conclude that they are stupid or deficient in some way and simply give up. The giving up may have the form of rebellion, aggressive behavior, defiance and the like, or simply withdrawal. And our prisons are overloaded with the casualties of this condition.

Moving on to F4 and F3, we see the Theta/Beta ratios are 2.94 at F4, which is the right frontal cortex, and 3.04 at F3, which is the left frontal cortex. Whenever we see elevated slow frequency or elevated Theta/Beta ratio over the sensory motor cortex (i.e., location Cz), we typically see it as well in the frontal cortex. Elevated Theta/Beta ratio in the frontal cortex is associated with hypoactivity of these regions of the brain and reflected in some inefficiency in cognitive processing.

So the first thing I know about this child is that he has a pernicious form of ADHD. In general, I know that the child has likely made efforts to try to pay attention and do his homework. However, he finds that no matter how hard he tries, the problems simply seem to get worse.

There are several other "flags" in Mitch's ClinicalQ that we will attend to shortly, but at this point I have enough information from the three circled areas (CZ, F3, and F4) to be able to discuss the situation with the child in front of me. So I say to, Mitch, "Mitch what the brain is telling me is that you have some problems staying focused in class. You find it difficult to pay attention, your mind tends to wander, and you have the same kind of problem when you try to do homework."

I now have Mitch's attention—he's focused on me. "But there is another thing in this record," I continue, "that's really problematic." "And it always causes students a lot of difficulty." "What the brain is telling me is that the harder you try the worse the situation gets." "No matter how hard you try, most of the time you find it extremely difficult to stay focused and on target both in class and when you are trying to do homework." "This is a problem we find mostly in men and it really makes you want to just give up!"

As is common at this point in my feedback to the child, Mitch is having difficulty maintaining composure. As I have been told by many children after their treatment is completed, they found that I was the "one person on the planet who understood" (to quote one recent client) what the situation was. They did not have to spend any time telling me what the problem was—I was able to see it from what the brain was telling me.

At this point I turned to Mitch's mother and asked if she would mind if I spoke with Mitch privately for a few moments. I often do this with teenage male clients for I find that it provides an opportunity for getting the child on board and committed to therapy. This is an opportunity to speak with the child without parents interrupting making comments and preventing me from developing good clinical attachment and report with the child.

In this particular case I noted several features of Mitch's brain assessment that made me suspicious about marijuana use. These indicators were elevated slow frequency Alpha and elevated slow frequency in the back of the brain under eyes-closed conditions. Very often you find this with individuals who are cannabis users. I decided to take a chance once I had developed some rapport with Mitch. Mitch and I spoke about the use of neurotherapy with professional sports teams and with the Canadian Olympic athletes. I then said: "Mitch it is important that you be part of your treatment team. I can help you with the brain inefficiencies that I see here in this brain map but it's important that you do what is necessary for these treatments to be really effective. And what I want you to do is stop smoking dope. Don't say 'yes' or 'no.' If you're not smoking dope so much the better but I'm getting some markers in your brain map that are often associated with cannabis use. If you are, stop because it makes people stupid. What cannabis does to people in your age range is it slows down a really important waveform in the brain and we certainly don't want that to happen."

As it turns out I was correct. Mitch was experimenting with marijuana. Mitch was so shaken by the accuracy of the brainwave assessment that I think he was shocked into stopping the marijuana use on the spot. We had a number of conversations and he shared with me later that he really felt like just quitting. He tearfully related that no matter how hard he tried, he simply could not function efficiently in school. He had great difficulty staying on target, doing his homework and not "looking stupid." He said he just couldn't wait until he could stop going to school. Neurotherapy saved this child's life, a sentiment expressed on several occasions by his mother.

This is the form of ADHD that, in my judgment, is the one form that is most represented in the statistics associated with ADHD and criminality. These are the kids that quit; these are the kids that become truant; these are the kids that act up in school; these are the kids that become marginalized; these are the kids that get themselves into trouble; and these are the kids that are associated with the statistics about the number of incarcerated youth that have the symptoms of ADHD.

So the 14-year-old young lad who came into my office in a sullen, bored, and clearly frightened state was indeed fortunate because the diagnosis and treatment of this child at this age clearly saved his life. Looking at the risk factors, it only makes sense to neurologically evaluate the condition of these children as soon as they run into difficulty in school. Teachers and parents are very aware of these behaviors very early in the child's life. The ease with which we can assess and diagnose the neurological anomalies is such that it is a tragedy that we are not doing so in our school systems.

Mitch is going on 20 at the time of this writing and is in the first few weeks of the third year of his undergraduate studies. Mitch had a total of 33 sessions between the ages of 14 and 16 and came back for a few more treatments when he felt that he was struggling at University.

The basic procedure at location Cz is to record ten 15-s epochs during which the client is engaged in specific activities. The client remains quietly observing the screen for two epochs following which there is one epoch of eyes closed. After epoch three the client's eyes are again open. It is important to be precise with the instruction to open and close the eyes. One wants to see rapid increase in Alpha and then sharp decrease in Alpha when the eyes are again opened. It is also important to watch the raw signal (or spectral display) to determine that the Alpha response is "healthy."

The remarkable clinical data ranges, such as ratios and summated bands, should be considered in the context of client variables such as age. For example, young children would be expected to have higher Theta/Beta ratios than adults. Hence, particular ratio levels are indicated as guidelines for the clinician to consider probing the client regarding a specific problem or characteristic. The basic clinical probes associated with the clinical norms are presented in this chapter. (The summary guide for administering the ClinicalQ and for the suggested clinical probes is found in Appendix A).

The raw data obtained from the ClinicalQ contains a wealth of information. The basic clinical probes provide the information for the intake session. As described by Susan Olding, it will allow surprisingly accurate identification of the problems for which the client is seeking treatment. However, there are many subtleties and nuances in the data set that will become apparent as one gains experience with "reading the Qs." In the following sections, in addition to the research supporting the clinical probes, some of the statistically significant nuances will be presented. These nuances often guide the clinician's formulation of a more textured conceptualization of the patient's situation.

Unremarkable Clinical Ranges

Location Cz At this location, three conditions are needed: Eyes open (EO), eyes closed (EC), and cognitive challenge (e.g., reading or counting backwards). In my clinic we also use this opportunity to determine the efficacy of some home treatment items such as harmonic sounds that influence brainwave activity. The OMNI Harmonic (Swingle 2010) that suppresses Theta amplitude, for example, is usually tested at location Cz.

Unremarkable clinical ranges for the measurements at Cz include: Theta/Beta ratio below 2.20 during EO and during cognitive challenge; Theta/SMR ratio below 3.00; the increase in Alpha band amplitude should be at least 30 % EC relative to EO; Alpha should block rapidly (i.e., drop to EO level quickly) so the post-EC epoch should be close to the pre-EC epoch Alpha amplitude if the Alpha blocking is efficient; TA (i.e., the sum of the amplitude of Theta, Alpha, and Beta bands) should be below 60.

Location O1 As most readers will surmise, the selection of location O1 reflects the legacy of Peniston's work on Alpha/Theta training (Peniston and Kulkosky 1999). At this location, the ClinicalQ is assessing the quietude of the CNS, the Alpha response, Alpha blocking, and excessively high, slow frequency amplitudes.

Unremarkable ranges are a Theta/Beta ratio between 1.80 and 2.20 both EO and EC, Alpha amplitude increase of at least 50 % EC relative to EO, return of Alpha amplitude to EO level within one epoch (i.e., the post-EC epoch is within 25 % of the pre-EC epoch amplitude), and TA below 60.

Locations F3 and F4 The ClinicalQ provides a wealth of information about behaviors from the assessment of the frontal cortex. Basically, the two locations should be balanced and the ratios among Theta, Alpha, and Beta to be symmetrical. The assessment of all frontal locations is done EC to reduce eye movement artifact problems. In my experience, a "rule-of-thumb" indicator of imbalance in the amplitudes in the frontal lobes is when the disparity is greater than about 15 %. However, as will be discussed below, we do find statistically significant differences in self-rated conditions when the disparity is 10 % or greater. These lower disparities may be conceptualized as shadow symptoms, but treatment of these imbalances is identical to those in the remarkable ranges.

In the frontal lobes, we want to see the amplitude of any brainwave band to be about the same at both F3 and F4. The unremarkable range would be that the difference between F3 and F4 in any band is less than 10 %. The Theta/Beta ratio is below 2.00 and the Theta/Alpha ratio is between 1.25 and 1.75. The TA is below 60.

Location Fz At this location, the ClinicalQ assesses the activity of the anterior cingulate gyrus, the Delta amplitude, and the ratio of Lo-Alpha to Hi-Alpha.

Normative ranges at location Fz are Delta below 9.0, the ratio of 28–40 Hz amplitude to Beta amplitude between 0.45 and 0.55, the sum of the latter two bands below 15, and the ratio of Lo-Alpha to Hi-Alpha below 1.50.

Remarkable Ranges

Sample Population

The ranges suggested as normative are based on more than three decades of clinical observation. There may be some slight differences in the ranges depending on the type of clinical EEG systems one is using. The ranges and threshold values, then, are offered as starting points to aid clinicians in identifying the EEG signatures that are associated with clinical symptoms.

On the first visit, every client completes a series of forms including various consent forms for treatment, authorization forms, basic biographical information forms, and two forms that ask about symptoms and behaviors. These forms are shown in the Appendices at the back of this book. The data for the statistical analyses presented throughout this manual are drawn from these intake questionnaires.

The statistical data presented below are offered to validate the robust features of the ClinicalQ. The sample consists of clients seen in my Vancouver clinic over the last several years. Only clients with complete data sets were included in the data sample. Further, only clients who did not designate a head injury or a condition that necessitated an initial full QEEG were included. The sample therefore excludes clients with epilepsy, traumatic brain injury, Parkinson's, stroke, Alzheimer's, and the like. The adult sample consists of 732 clients. The child sample consists of 547 clients.

Specialty populations include seniors, over 80 years old ($N=30$); left handed ($N=110$); independently diagnosed (by psychiatrist) bipolar ($N=37$); Sleep disordered with four-night EEG monitoring ($N=52$). All samples are combined gender—no clinical benefit has been found for independent gender norms. Unless otherwise noted, all probabilities are based on 2-tail statistical distributions.

Clinical Implications of Remarkable Ranges

The above normative ranges were established from data collected on clinical populations. The normative values will vary as a function of many variables such as time of day, medication/drug history, physiological state of the client, and client age, to name but a few.

The reader may note that these normative values are far more stringent than those of the normative databases. Further, studies comparing clinical populations versus nonclinical populations (e.g., ADHD vs. nonclinical comparison group) find normative discriminative ranges that are considerably higher than some of the normative ranges of the ClinicalQ. The reason for this is obvious. Clients come to a neurotherapist complaining, for example, of problems with attention and focus. Relative to their own EEG, one may find that the only area showing any elevation is in the excess of Theta amplitude, reflected in the Theta/Beta ratio, over the sensory motor cortex (location Cz). This elevation may seem minimal with a ratio in the low 2 plus range. In any controlled study, comparing this person with a group of nonclinical cohorts, a ratio of that magnitude would probably not be statistically different from the control group mean. However, that does not mean that this is not the brain condition associated with this client's complaint of problems with attention. One client with a Theta/Beta ratio of 2.50 at location Cz may not complain of any problems with focus and hence they do not appear in the neurotherapist's office. Another person with exactly the same ratio, on the other hand, may seek treatment for attention problems and find that the condition improves when the ratio is reduced. In short, the remarkable ranges are clinical heuristic ranges. Whether or not they survive discriminative function statistical comparisons with nonclinical groups is largely irrelevant. One should always keep in mind that the client is sitting in the neurotherapist's office because he or she has a troublesome symptom. The beneficial feature of the ClinicalQ is that one can isolate areas of brain activity that may be associated with the symptom even if the activity is not statistically different from a nonclinical group normative range.

Symptoms Associated with Remarkable Ranges at Location Cz

Two and one half minutes of recording at location Cz provides the neurotherapist with a wealth of valuable information. First, one looks at the overall Theta/Beta ratio. Ideally, we want to see that ratio below 2 or so. If the ratio is above 2.20, probe the client to determine if focus and attention are a problem. Even if the overall, or mean, ratio is below 2.20 but one finds that under cognitive challenge (e.g., reading, counting) the ratio goes above 2.20, also probe for attention problems.

From our clinical sample, of the 39 children who were rated by a parent as "hyperactive" (4 or 5 on a five-point scale), 71.8 % had Theta/Beta ratios above 2.20 and 28.2 % had ratios below 2.20 ($z = 4.27$, $p < 0.001$, $N = 39$). Sixty-seven children from our sample were rated by a parent as 4 or 5 on the item "attention problems in school." From this sample, 70.2 % had a Theta/Beta ratio above 2.20 and 29.8 % had ratios below 2.20 ($z = 5.11$, $p < 0.001$, $N = 67$). The finding of elevated Theta/Beta ratios in clients diagnosed with ADHD is quite robust. Thompson and Thompson (2006), Chabot et al. (2001), and Barry et al. (2006) likewise report that a large proportion (around 80 %) of clients diagnosed with ADHD show this elevated Theta/Beta ratio pattern. Even minor elevation in the Theta/Beta ratio (above 2.30) results in a highly reliable increase in the average rating on the "problems with concentration" question (difference = 6.1 %, $N = 631$, $t = 4.45$, $p < 0.001$) and "…often do not remember what I have just read" question (difference = 3.8 %, $N = 635$, $t = 2.35$, $p < 0.02$).

If the Theta/Beta ratio jumps substantially (25 % or greater) under a cognitive challenge, such as reading, then probe to determine if the client frequently experiences reading a paragraph and then discovering that they cannot remember what they had just read. In my experience, one usually gets an affirmative reply to that query.

From our adult database, 59 clients' intake data showed at least a 15 % jump in the Theta/Beta ratio under reading condition. Of that sample, 6.8 % rated themselves as not experiencing problems with remembering what they have just read whereas 45.8 % of this sample of adults rated themselves high on this same questionnaire item ($z = 5.34$, $p < 0.001$, $N = 59$).

It appears that this form of ADHD, when the Theta/Beta increases under cognitive challenge, is a particularly pernicious form. Experience with many clients gives the clinical impression of greater struggle and discouragement with academic work. One gets the impression of children, in particular, wanting to just give up and quit because "the harder they try the worse the condition gets," a statement that always seems to resonate with these children. It is important to also note that, at rest, this condition is frequently missed because the ratios remain within normal range. It is only when the child is cognitively challenged with reading or a mental math task that the condition manifests.

Related findings seem relevant here. Parent rating of "easily frightened" is related to the Theta/Beta ratio under challenge. Children rated, by a parent, as "easily frightened" had an, under challenge, Theta/Beta ratio that was, on average, 10 % greater than the at rest ratio ($t = 2.33$, $p = 0.02$, $df = 143$). This relationship between fear and the Theta/Beta ratio was not found for the at rest condition. Also, children rated as "Stubborn" had under challenge Theta/Beta ratios that were, on average, 15 % greater than those rated low on this trait ($t = 5.60$, $p < 0.001$, $df = 162$). This relationship also was not significant under at rest conditions.

If the Theta/Beta ratio remains relatively constant between rest and cognitive challenge but one observes that the Beta has increased substantially (greater than 25 %) between these two conditions, then probe the client to determine if they find reading fatiguing. Often we find that the Theta amplitude increases substantially under cognitive challenge, but this increase is not reflected in an increased Theta/Beta ratio because of a simultaneous increase in Beta amplitude. It appears as though the client is compensating for the Theta amplitude increase by increasing mental effort. This condition can also result from eye problems in which eyestrain is causing an EMG artifact resulting in increased amplitudes for both Beta and Theta.

If the Theta/Beta ratio is below 2.20 on average but well above that value when reading, this could be either ADD or have problems with comprehension/retention of information. Often, of course, it is both of these conditions. However, one does encounter clients for whom attention in class does not seem to be a major problem, but the children have considerable difficulties in comprehension and/or retention of written material.

Another condition that also is often associated with poor retention of written material is when the Alpha response is blunted or absent. The increase in Alpha amplitude should be at least 30 % between eyes open and eyes closed. When the Alpha response is deficient, clients often complain of poor retention of information and/or poor short-term memory. On the simple question of "I am forgetful" clients with an Alpha response below 15 % at Cz had an average response 8 % higher (more forgetful) as compared with clients with Alpha responses above 35 % ($t=2.36$, $df=640$, $p<0.02$). Those with an Alpha response greater than 35 % were more than twice as likely to rate themselves as having no problem at all with forgetfulness (1 on the 5-point scale) as compared with those with an Alpha response below 15 % ($z=2.59$, $p<0.01$, $N=643$). Conversely, those rating themselves as forgetful (4 or 5 on the 5-point scale) versus those who rated themselves as not forgetful (1) had an Alpha response that was, on average, 28.2 % lower in amplitude ($t=2.06$, $p=0.04$, $df=380$).

Slow return of the Alpha response (Alpha amplitude return to eyes-open level following eyes-closed condition) was related to children's "sleep disturbances" as rated by a parent. The Alpha amplitude level of the sleep disturbed rated child was 117.6 % greater than the child without a sleep problem ($t=2.12$, $p<0.04$, $df=166$). This could indicate that the sleep disturbed child has a problem shutting off visual images or perhaps more difficulty in state changes. Although no data are available, clinical impression also suggests that some individuals with a history of emotional trauma also show slow Alpha returns as well.

When the Alpha response is blunted or negative (i.e., the Alpha amplitude is lower under eyes-closed condition than under eyes-open condition) then one should consider the possibility of traumatic stress (Swingle 2001, 2013). If the Alpha response is negative at both locations Cz and O1, there is a strong likelihood that the client has experienced or is experiencing emotionally traumatic conditions.

I became aware of this trauma signature when working with clients with Posttraumatic Stress Disorder (PTSD) at McLean Hospital. These traumatized clients included Vietnam veterans and police officers, among others. It became obvious during the ClinicalQ that these clients had no Alpha response at Cz and/or O1. There were a few exceptions, as will be discussed below, but the vast majority of the clients that I treated showed this deficit. Metaphorically, one can conceptualize this as the brain protecting itself against the major stressor of PTSD, the flashbacks. Alpha being a visualization response, it is intuitively consistent that this dampened Alpha response would be reinforced by fear or avoidance.

If the Alpha response is negative at Cz but present at O1, then one occasionally finds that the client experiences memory and retention difficulties but does not admit to traumatic stress. In addition, when the blunting is only found at Cz, the emotionally stressing situation is more likely to be current or recent. Blunting that only appears at O1, on the other hand, is more likely to be associated with historical traumatic events. Again, these generalizations offer hypotheses for the clinician to probe with the client. However, as will be discussed latter in this book, these subtleties can offer remarkable insight into understanding the conditions that are affecting the client.

For example, in the Clinic, we often encounter children who have been referred for treatment of AD(H)D who show no EEG anomalies associated with attention or focus problems, but show the trauma signature. Proceeding cautiously, we probe for past or present emotionally traumatic stress. We have encountered a number of cases in which the child's attention and focus problems were stress related and not a function of any AD(H)D brain pattern. Several examples of recent cases include bullying, hospital experiences, serious parental illness, sexual abuse, and family violence. Later in this book many such cases will be reviewed.

As one would expect, individuals with these trauma markers frequently report depressed and/or anxious mood states. From our database, clients who rated themselves at level 4 or 5 (on a five-point scale) on "I feel depressed" had Alpha responses almost 50 % lower in amplitude on average (48.8 μV vs. 72.4 μV; $n=346$, $t=3.09$, $p<0.004$) as compared to those rating themselves at a 1 ("Not true of me"). Those rating themselves at 4 or 5 on "I am very anxious" had an Alpha response that on average was 27.3 % lower in amplitude (51.6 μV vs. 65.7 μV; $n=437$, $t=2.14$, $p<0.04$) than those rating themselves at a 1.

There are many issues that must be addressed with respect to how one should proceed when the trauma signature is encountered. First, is it really trauma? We have encountered situations with both adults and children in which the clients were not aware of, or did not admit to, any trauma. In my experience this is relatively uncommon, although we have encountered clients with severe learning disorders, and markedly blunted Alpha, who are adamant that trauma was not part of their history.

Second, and most importantly, is the neurotherapist competent to deal with trauma and, if not, is the neurotherapist properly networked to refer the client to a competent person? Neurotherapy is not a stand-alone discipline and nowhere is this more apparent than in the case of trauma. Neurotherapists without adequate psychological training should not handle cases of this nature. At best, the client is not going to improve much, because a major cause of the client's difficulties is left unaddressed. At worst, the client is going to abreact with a neurotherapist not equipped to deal with problems of this severity.

Drawing examples from our adult database, when the Alpha response is below 10 % at both Cz and O1, over 80 % admit to having a history of emotional trauma ($z=4.40$, $p<0.001$, $N=54$). The situation is not as clear when dealing with individuals with a strong Alpha response, such as a person with strong visualization skills (the artist signature).

Strong Alpha response at both locations Cz and O1 has been shown to be related to clients rating themselves as "artistic." Clients with Alpha responses above 80 % rated themselves as high on the "I am very artistic" questions, 47.3 % more often than clients with Alpha response below 25 % ($z = 2.86$, $p < 0.005$, $N = 591$). Clients rating themselves high on the artistic question (4 or 5) had an Alpha response that was 26.1 % stronger, on average, as compared with clients who rate themselves at a 1 level ($t = 2.08$, $p < 0.04$, $N = 415$). This "artists' signature" is also found at location O1 as will be discussed later. It is interesting to note that those clients rating themselves as high on the artistic question tend to have higher Theta/Beta ratios at location Cz under eyes open ($M = 8.9$ % higher, $t = 2.66$, $p < 0.01$) and reading conditions ($M = 8.2$ %, $t = 2.33$, $p < 0.02$).

When clients have strong resident Alpha (e.g., artists), the blunting effect of trauma can be obscured in the summary statistics. Skilled neurotherapists can see trauma on a strong Alpha response because of the unique patterning. The "traumatized artist signature" on the raw signal or EEG single hertz spectral display has the look of the Alpha amplitude being "pushed down." It is also frequently found that current exposure to severe emotional stressors with clients who have the artist's strong Alpha response will show blunting at Cz and much less so at O1. This was the pattern observed in the previously discussed case of the child who was being bullied at school. His Alpha response at location Cz was about 19 % whereas at O1 it was nearly 100 %.

A related finding also suggests that the blunted Alpha response is related to exposure to emotional trauma and further that this exposure may have effects on the child's sense of security. Children whose parents rated them as "easily frightened" had an average Alpha response of 27.6 % (below the clinical threshold for trauma marker) as compared with an average response of 49.5 % for children rated as not easily frightened ($t = 3.39$, $p < 0.001$, $df = 152$). This is directly relevant to the issue of causes other than ADHD that effect a child's academic performance. They may just be afraid, hypervigilant, or insecure which in turn affects their ability to focus and be attentive in school. The case of the child with a ClinicalQ profile suggesting that he may have been the victim of bullying, discussed in this book, is a good example of a situation in which a frightened child was assumed to have ADHD when in fact the fear was a primary cause of his problems with focus.

Two cases of clients who experienced serious trauma during the time of their treatment with us show how trauma suppresses the Alpha response. Both of these clients had strong Alpha responses, and both rated themselves as having good artistic skills on our intake questionnaires. In one case, a young child found a dead body while playing in a wooded area, and the second case was a young woman whose best friend committed suicide just one day before we remapped her Alpha response. In the first situation, the Alpha response was reduced by 69.4 % after the trauma. The treatment for this condition, in addition to counseling, is to "release" the Alpha response with neurotherapy and/or emotional release therapies including EMDR, somatoemotional release, hypnosis, and the like (Swingle 2006, April). In this case, neurotherapy was all that was required, in addition to the counseling. After three neurotherapy sessions of Alpha increase at Cz and O1, the Alpha response was restored to within 12 % of the pre-trauma level. In the second case mentioned above, this 20-year-old young woman learned of the suicide of her best friend just one day before the brain assessment. The Alpha suppression was 21.9 % in one location and 46.5 % in the second location.

Research from the Swingle Clinic (Swingle 2013) indicated that the Alpha response could be blunted with brief exposures to strong emotionally negative photographs. Clients viewed either no pictures, a positive picture (horse and farmer in a field), or a negative photo (dead body being dragged with an ice hook on the skull in Nazi concentration camp) for 10 s. The Alpha response taken before viewing the pictures (or no picture control) was compared with a second Alpha response after the experimental condition. The negative photo resulted in an average Alpha response blunting of −62.3 %. The positive photo and no photo viewed conditions both resulted in the second Alpha response being greater than the first (no photo = +33.3 %; positive photo = +108.9 %; (all comparisons with negative photo, $p < 0.0005$).

It is interesting that clients occasionally seem to be unaware of their traumatic history. Startling examples include a family in which I found the trauma signature in the map of a 14-year-old boy. The father, who was present during the assessment, stated that he was not aware of any trauma that his son "was not dealing with well." The latter type of statement is usually a "red flag," so I pushed the father about issues the boy was coping with. It turns out that the boy's uncle had been murdered 2 weeks prior to the assessment.

Another example is when a client seems to be unaware of a trauma but after a while "recalls" the event which is usually reported at a subsequent visit. In one such case, an 81-year-old man had an Alpha response of 20.9 % at Cz and negative 2.4 % at O1 but maintained that he was unaware of any emotional trauma history. After six neurotherapy treatments, his Alpha responses were 32 % at Cz and 31.7 % at O1. At the sixth session, he reported that he "suddenly" remembered two horrific traumas that had occurred during wartime. Such spontaneous recall of trauma occurs quite frequently when the Alpha response is restored, either with neurotherapy or with some other procedures such as EMDR, hypnosis, bilateral somatosensory stimulation, somatoemotional release, and the like.

There also appears to be a mild relationship between SMR amplitude and artistic self-ratings. Clients rating themselves high on "artistic" had an average SMR amplitude that was 14.8 % stronger than clients rating themselves as 1 on the artistic question ($t = 2.24$, $p < 0.03$, $df = 76$). However, based on the seminal research of Dr. Sterman, the principal issue associated with SMR amplitude training is body quieting. As discussed throughout this book, SMR training is a very effective procedure for treating seizure disorders, headache, muscular restlessness, and involuntary movement conditions.

Clients who rate themselves low on "restless and cannot sit still" have, on average, 11.7 % higher SMR amplitude as compared with clients rating themselves high on this factor ($t = 2.03$, $df = 72$, $p < 0.05$). In addition, those clients with rating themselves high on restlessness had ratios of Theta/Beta to SMR amplitude that was, on average, 57.5 % greater than those rating themselves low on this factor ($z=3.02$, $N=172$, $p<0.003$). Those who rate themselves low on "tired and fatigued" have an SMR amplitude that is, on average, 14.3 % higher than those rating themselves low on this factor ($t=1.93$, $df=96$, $p<0.06$).

Two features often observed with clients who show elevated Total Amplitude (TA) are feelings of fatigue and cognitive inefficiencies. TA is defined as the summation of the amplitude in microvolts of Theta, Alpha, and Beta. The metaphor that comes to mind when observing these clients with elevated TA is that the brain is working hard but inefficiently. In my clinical experience, I see this elevated TA more frequently with clients with developmental delay, intellectual compromise, traumatic brain injury, and often with fibromyalgia. As compared with clients with TA below 40.0, those above 60.0 rated themselves as 20.4 % higher on the "I feel tired and fatigued most of the time" question ($t=4.74$, $df=639$, $p<0.001$) and 10.8 % higher on the "I often do not remember what I have just read" question ($t=2.42$, $df=643$, $p<0.02$) (Table 2.2).

Symptoms Associated with Remarkable Ranges at Position O1

Historically, brainwave biofeedback was fixated on location Cz, and there are some interesting reasons for this choice (Berger 1969). However, if I were forced to select only one site for an assessment, I would unhesitantly select an occipital site such as O1. The information one can obtain from a one-minute recording of just the three bandwidths of Alpha, Theta, and Beta is indeed extensive.

First, as described in the section on remarkable features at location Cz, above, if one finds an absence of the Alpha response then trauma or significant emotional turmoil is decidedly probable. The increase in Alpha amplitude from eyes closed to eyes open should be at least 50 % at location O1. If it is low or negative, then emotional trauma is likely. Clinically, it appears as though Alpha blunting at Cz but not at O1 is indicative of a current emotional stressing situation, such as bullying. Blunting at O1, on the other hand, appears to be associated with historical trauma. Often one sees the blunting at both locations. The agreement rate, that is when a client admits to either a history of traumatic stress or current severe emotional stress, when the ClinicalQ shows Alpha blunting at Cz, O1, or both is well over 90 %. Marked blunting of Alpha at location O1 is a cardinal marker with clients diagnosed with PTSD.

If the Alpha response is much higher, say 150 %, then I usually ask the client about artistic interest or skills. Such artistic interests can include the visual arts, dance, poetry, construction (e.g., model building), and the like. The strong Alpha response is not particularly common, at least in our clinical research population. Selecting those clients who rated themselves as high on "artistic" on the intake questionnaire, 36 % had strong Alpha responses of at least 75 % at Cz and 150 % at O1. Of the 49 clients who rated themselves as having no artistic skill, 20.4 % had Alpha responses that exceeded the above criteria. This difference is statistically

Table 2.2 Basic clinical probes for location Cz

Formula Amplitude in microvolts (μV)	Norms	Remarkable range	Clinical implication probe
Alpha response			
Alpha(EC) – Alpha(EO)/Alpha(EC)	>30 %	<30 % or negative	If <30 % or negative, ask about visual processing (memory) problem; poor retention of information and/or poor short term memory; exposure to severe emotional stressor; also refer to O1 Alpha Response % change
Alpha recovery			
Alpha(EO) – Alpha(EO) after/ Alpha(EC) before	<25 %	>25 %	If >25 %, ask about foggy thinking; older clients ask about cognitive decline, sleep problems, medications; younger clients probe sleep deprivation, marijuana
Theta(EC)/SMR(EC)	<3.0	>3.0	If >3.0, ask about inability to sit still or quiet the body; sleep disturbance as in trouble falling asleep
			If >3.0, ask about problems related to muscle activity such as headaches, chronic pain, body tremors, dystonia, and seizure disorders that have a motor component
Theta(EO)/Beta(EO)	<2.2	>2.2	If >2.2, ask about CADD to see if focus and attention are a problem; also refer to T/B (UT) description
Theta(UT)/Beta(UT)	<2.2	>2.2	If >2.2, ask about CADD; ratio should drop under task when compared to eyes open
			If >2.2 and if Theta(EO)/Beta(EO) < 2.2, ask about ADD and/or problems with poor reading comprehension/retention and getting tired when reading
		>3.0	If >3.0, ask about ADHD
Beta(EO) – Beta(UT)/Beta(EO)	<15 %	>15 %	If >15 %, ask about getting overly tired when reading or problem solving
T/B (EO) – T/B (UT)/T/B(EO)	<15 %	>15 %	If >15 %, ask about CADD
Theta Omni % change			
Theta(Omni) – Theta(EO)/Theta(EC)			If positive %, Theta increased with Omni sound, do not prescribe for home use
			If negative with Omni sound, prescribe for home use
Total amplitude (EC)			
Theta(EC) + Alpha(EC) + Beta(EC)	<60	>60	If >60, ask about development delay, autistic spectrum behavior, marked cognitive deficits
Peak alpha frequency (EC)	>9.5	<9.5	If <9.5, ask about mental sluggishness
Peak alpha frequency (EO)	>9.5	<9.5	If <9.5, ask about mental sluggishness

significant ($z=2.66$, $p<0.01$, $N=99$). However, given that this is a clinical population, it is likely that some clients with artistic skill may also have experienced an emotional trauma that would suppress the strong Alpha response. Those rating themselves high on artistic had an Alpha response that was 31.9 % stronger than those rating themselves as low on this dimension ($t=2.56$, $p=0.01$, $df=413$). Also, those who rated themselves as high on artistic had stronger Theta/Beta ratios, both eyes open (8 %, $t=2.12$, $p<0.04$, $df=414$) and eyes closed (9.5 %, $t=2.40$, $p<0.02$, $df=413$), compared with those rating themselves low on this trait.

Since artistic skill is often associated with a strong Alpha response, then a blunted Alpha response could also reflect trauma. One can often see this on the EEG spectral display during the intake ClinicalQ, provided the data are in real time and not statistically distorted, such as running averages. What one observes is that when the eyes are closed, the Alpha will jump and then will start to rapidly decline, looking much like something pushing down on the amplitude. One can also observe this pattern of blunted Alpha response with traumatized clients who have partially resolved the trauma through psychotherapy. I reported on several such cases (Swingle 2002, February) in which emotional integration techniques (e.g., EMDR, somatoemotional release, and hypnosis) that had been successful resulted in restoration of the Alpha response and increase in the Theta/Beta ratio. Changes in the opposite direction also occur, of course, such as emotional abreaction to release of the Alpha response and/or increase of Theta amplitude. Qualified psychotherapists can utilize this emotional reaction to dramatically accelerate the therapeutic processing of the traumatic content. There are some learning disorders that mimic the trauma brainwave profile in that, in addition to some other brainwave anomalies, there is the absence of an Alpha response at both Cz and O1.

The "artist's signature" mentioned above is the opposite of the trauma profile. In this case, the Alpha amplitude increase EC relative to EO is about threefold at Cz and fourfold at O1. If baseline Alpha is high, then these increases may be somewhat less. Basically, the artist's signature reflects the ability to visualize and manifests in artistic interest and skill. This skill may be in the visual arts such as painting or sculpture, construction such as carpentry or model building, architecture, poetry, fiction writing, or dance and choreography. Engaging a reluctant child in the neurotherapeutic process is always made easier when I find the artist's signature because inevitably the child and the child's parents will enthusiastically admit to such skills. I then emphasize that this is a most valuable gift and proceed to elaborate on how this unique skill will help the child to succeed in various occupations.

It is also interesting to note that clients who report that "Sometimes I cannot get rid of annoying or disturbing thoughts" have an Alpha response that is, on average, 31.2 % stronger than those rating themselves low on this dimension ($t=2.10$, $p<0.04$, $df=430$). It is essential for the neurotherapist to monitor the raw EEG signal when recording the Alpha response. Those with strong Alpha amplitude baselines show identifiable Alpha blunting patterns associated with exposure to emotional stress, which are often obscured in the averages because of the strong Alpha amplitude baseline. Strong visualization skills could well be associated with perseveration of annoying emotional thoughts. Informing the client of the possibility of artistic skill being related to the perseveration of emotional thoughts can often be helpful in that the client understands the pluses as well as potential negatives of any departure from normative brain functioning.

The increased perseveration in thought processes that may be associated with a strong Alpha response can also have a positive effect in terms of increased retention of information. Clients who rate themselves high on "I often do not remember what I have just read" have an Alpha response that is, on average, 26.4 % lower than those rating themselves as low on this factor ($t=2.13$, $p<0.04$, $df=418$). In addition, those who rate themselves high on "forgetful" have an Alpha response that is 34.4 % lower than those rating themselves low on this attribute ($t=2.84$, $p<0.005$, $df=380$).

The second critical metric is the Theta/Beta ratio. In the back of the brain, we want to see this ratio between about 1.80 and 2.20. The low Theta/Beta ratio can be associated with inadequate Theta amplitude, excessive Beta amplitude, or both. From a neurotherapeutic perspective, the nature of the inadequate ratio is not important other than determining the training thresholds for Theta and Beta amplitudes. However, clinically one often notes differences in the client's demeanor depending on whether the Theta is low as opposed to the Beta being high.

Deficiencies in the Theta/Beta ratio in this region of the brain are associated with the brain being inefficient in self-quieting. The client finds it difficult to find "peace in their head," to quote a recent client. Low Theta/Beta ratio is associated with poor stress tolerance, racing thoughts, inability to "shut the brain off," general anxiety, self-medicating and/or distraction oriented behaviors, burnout-based depression, and problems with sleep quality.

Only 18 % of clients from our database who rated their anxiety as a "one" on the five-point scale had Theta/Beta ratios below 1.40, whereas 62 % of clients who stated that they were seeking treatment for anxiety had a Theta/Beta ratio below 1.40 ($z=6.98$, $p<0.001$, $N=97$). Clients who rate themselves high on "I am very anxious" have, on average, a 24.4 % (eyes open) and a 22.9 % (eyes closed) lower Theta/Beta ratio relative to those clients who rate themselves as not anxious (eyes open: $t=5.92$, $p<0.0001$, $df=437$; eyes closed: $t=5.48$, $p<0.0001$, $df=436$).

Clients who rate themselves high on "depression" have, on average, a 41.4 % lower amplitude (eyes open) and a 40.2 % lower (eyes closed) Theta/Beta ratio at location O1 relative to those clients who rate themselves not depressed (eyes open: $t=7.34$, $p<0.0001$, $df=245$; eyes closed: $t=8.62$, $p<0.0001$, $df=244$). In addition, the correlation between the ratings of "I feel depressed" and "I am very anxious" is 0.51 ($p<0.0001$, $df=901$) indicating that many clients who report depression may well be experiencing the sequellae of severe anxiety without any of the neurological markers for depression. Clients with Theta/Beta ratios below 1.00 have, on average, 12.0 % higher ratings on "I feel depressed" relative to those with Theta/Beta ratios above 1.50 ($t=3.03$, $p=0.003$, $df=753$). Clients who rate themselves high on "I have a positive emotional life" also have a Theta/Beta ratio that, on average, is 9.4 % greater than those rating themselves very low on this characteristic ($t=2.08$, $p<0.04$, $df=374$).

Of 14 self-designated alcoholics and drug addicts drawn from the client data sample, 13 (92.8 %) had a Theta/Beta ratio below 1.40 as measured at location O1.

Compared with the previous samples of clients rating themselves high versus low on the anxiety questionnaire item, 18.2 % of clients rating themselves low in anxiety had a Theta/Beta ratio below 1.40 ($z=5.52$, $p<0.002$, $N=25$) and 62.0 % of clients rating themselves high in anxiety had ratio below 1.40 ($z=3.58$, $p<0.002$, $N=100$). Thus, even compared with clients rating themselves as very high in anxiety, a significantly greater proportion of self-designated alcoholics/addicts had the low Theta/Beta ratios.

Elevated Beta amplitude in alcoholics has also been noted at other locations other than O1. Rangaswamy et al. (2002), for example, report that most of the Beta bands are elevated over much of the brain in alcoholics. Maurage et al. (2008) report disturbed processing of anger in alcoholics, at both behavioral and electrophysiological levels. Sakusic et al. (2010) report that in a study of veterans with PTSD, significant correlations were found between alcohol usage and state and trait of anger, angry temperament, anger expression, and anger control. PTSD hyperarousal symptoms were significantly correlated to state anger and use of alcohol. In our clinical database, 435 clients (from total of 834) had a Theta/Beta ratio below 1.2 at location O1. Of that group, 38 (8.7 %) rated themselves as not having an anger problem, whereas 134 (30.8 %) rated themselves high on this factor ($z=8.9$, $p<0.001$, $N=172$).

A low Theta/Beta ratio in the occipital region is an indication that the brain is inefficient in self-restoration, so the client often reports vulnerability to colds, flus, and the like. I also believe that this may be a predisposing condition for Posttraumatic Stress Disorder, fibromyalgia, chronic fatigue, essential exhaustion, and severe withdrawal problems when discontinuing medications like the benzodiazepines.

Although a low Theta/Beta ratio (e.g., below 1.40 or so, either eyes-open or eyes-closed) is often found with clients who report sleep quality problems, there is a specific marker that is usually associated with problems with sleep onset and/or regaining sleep after mid-sleep awakenings. That marker is when the eyes-closed Theta/Beta ratio is noticeably less than the eyes-open ratio. Several factors are important, such as the overall level of the Theta/Beta ratios. If the ratios are very low under both eyes-open and eyes-closed conditions, then sleep disturbance is likely and the specific marker is less likely to be apparent. However, when one finds that the ratio under eyes open is above about 1.50, then a disparity of 25 % or so between eyes-open and eyes-closed may be meaningful.

In general, those admitting to sleep problems have an average eyes-closed Theta/Beta ratio that is 8 % lower than those rating themselves as having no sleep problems ($t=2.06$, $p=0.04$, $df=465$). And for those rating themselves as having sleep problems, the eyes-closed Theta/Beta ratio is 20 % lower than the eyes-open ratio ($t=6.80$, $p<0.0001$, $df=706$). The lower eyes-closed relative to eyes-open Theta/Beta ratio is the cardinal marker for sleep disturbance. ClinicalQ markers specific to deficiencies in specific sleep phases are discussed in the next chapter.

For children, those whose parents rated as having sleep problems had, on average, an eyes-closed Theta/Beta ratio that was 10.6 % lower than those rated as not having sleep problems ($t=1.97$, $p<0.05$, $df=183$). It is also interesting to note that children whose parents rated as having a problem with retention of information show a 14 % lower Theta/Beta ratio, both eyes-open and eyes-closed, as compared with children rated as having no information retention difficulties (eyes-open: $t=2.54$, $p=0.01$, $df=164$; eyes-closed: $t=2.30$, $p=0.02$, $df=154$). In addition, children parentally rated as "unhappy" had, on average, 18 % lower Theta/Beta ratio eyes-open ($t=2.95$, $p<0.004$, $df=135$) and 22.8 % lower ratio eyes-closed ($t=3.43$, $p<0.001$, $df=129$). The relationship between low Theta/Beta ratio and unhappiness in children may reflect mood factors associated with fatigue, lack of sleep, or poor stress tolerance and anxiety. Children with lower Theta/Beta ratios both eyes-open and eyes-closed are rated as "indifferent" by parents. (eyes open: $t=1.92$, $p<0.06$, $df=142$; eyes-closed: $t=2.92$, $p<0.005$, $df=136$). This may be related to depression in that young children with depressed mood states often do not present as sad but as disinterested and unmotivated. As well, this finding is consistent with the previously reported relationship to parental ratings of "unhappy." Also consistent, parental ratings of "poor self-esteem" are likewise associated with low Theta/Beta ratio at this occipital location ($t=2.01$, $p<0.05$, $df=139$). As would be expected, children with low Theta/Beta ratios are less stress tolerant and more vulnerable to illness as indicated by parental rating of "frequently ill" ($t=2.01$, $p<0.05$, $df=199$). These children are also rated, by a parent, as more "easily frightened" (difference = 12.5 %, $t=1.99$, $p<0.05$, $df=151$). As will be reviewed later in this book, depressed mood state is often associated with anxiety and fatigue, which may be the result of the low Theta/Beta ratio.

Drawing from our database, we selected clients who rated themselves as having no sleep problems at all versus those who identified sleep disturbance as a reason for seeking treatment. From the database, 92 clients indicated that they had no sleep issues at all and 90 indicated that a sleep problem was a reason for seeking treatment. The clients were further selected for those who had an eyes-closed Theta/Beta ratio that was at least 25 % less than their eyes-open ratio. Of the sample of 182 clients, 60 % in the sleep disturbed group had eyes-closed Theta/Beta ratios at least 25 % below the eyes-open ratio as compared with 37 % of those in the no sleep disturbed group. The test of the difference in proportions indicated a significant difference between the two groups ($z=4.20$, $p<0.001$, $N=182$). Deficient Theta/Beta ratios at the O1 location indicate that the patient is likely to admit to some form of sleep disturbance. The deficient ratio does not indicate the nature of the sleep disturbance which can vary considerably including issues associated with sleep onset insomnia, frequent awakenings, inability to regain sleep after wakening, inadequate REM sleep, and inadequate Deep Sleep. The relationship of the ClinicalQ to sleep architecture is discussed in detail in the following chapter.

When the client admits to some sleep disturbance when questioned based on the deficiency in the Theta/Beta ratios, the clinician generally will further question the client regarding sleep hygiene matters. Although we tend to presume that sleep disturbance may well be associated with poor sleep hygiene, it is always worth keeping in mind that neurological factors affecting sleep quality may result in poor sleep hygiene habits rather than the other way around. So, for example, an individual who experiences difficulty falling asleep may develop the habit of staying up late to become fatigued to enable sleep.

It is important at this point to repeat that the above ranges are clinical normative ranges. People manage quite well in life, I presume, with Theta/Beta ratios well below 1.80. However, when a client presents for treatment, departures from these clinically derived normative values identify behavior patterns that are problematic for that client. Hence, the scientific philosophy is quite different in that one is not concerned with a value that is two or three standard deviations beyond a statistical average, but rather, is the metric in question remarkable in the context of that client's ClinicalQ. If a client presents with a ClinicalQ that satisfies all of the normative ranges except at O1 where the ratio is modestly below normative (say 1.60), then I venture the supposition, to the client, that they experience some of the above-mentioned symptoms. If they support the supposition, which they routinely do, then we can rapidly proceed to treatment to correct the problems.

It is equally important to note that this clinical profile would likely have been completely missed if the neurotherapist had relied on a normative database discrimination because the ratio would have survived statistical cutoffs based on mean deviations. Further, we are likely to be able to treat this problem at a cost that is perhaps only a bit more than this client would have been charged for just a "traditional" intake assessment and follow-up. As with any normative range, the more marked the departure, the more likely that the client will admit to more of the symptoms and the symptoms are likely to be more severe. The observant clinician will notice that there are some interesting qualitative differences between clients with excessive Beta amplitude and those with deficient Theta amplitude even though the resultant Theta/Beta ratios are about the same.

Too much Theta amplitude relative to Beta amplitude is an indicator of interpersonal detachment with the qualitative character of autistic/Asperger's behavior. Such ratios tend to be above 3.00 before we see frank autistic-like presentation; however, even at lower levels, one often hears client's report that their intimate associates complain of such detachment. This detachment, in combination with other deficiencies that were more likely the reason for the client presenting for treatment, can be negatively synergic. An example of this negative synergy would be when a client has a disparity in the frontal lobes, associated with depression (discussed below) and the above condition predisposing to detachment. In this case, the client would strongly benefit not only from neurotherapy to equalize frontal lobe activity but also treatment to reduce the Theta/Beta ratio in the occipital region of the brain.

A condition we frequently encounter is that of clients who have been incorrectly treated for depression when the problem is anxiety. Clients with severe anxiety conditions often feel hopeless and out of control and define that condition as depression. This is often misdiagnosed and the client then is medicated with antidepressants which prove to be ineffective. These clients often have no neurological indicators of depression but one or more markers for poor stress tolerance, anxiety, or perseverative thought processes. One of the markers for poor stress tolerance is the deficient Theta/Beta ratio at location O1. Clients with deficient Theta/Beta ratio are more likely to rate themselves as depressed. The rating of "I feel depressed" was 12 % higher on average for clients with Theta/Beta ratio below 1.00 compared with those with a ratio of 1.50 ($t=3.03$, $df=435$, $p<0.005$). These conditions will be addressed more thoroughly later in this chapter (Table 2.3).

Table 2.3 Basic clinical probes for location O1

Formula Amplitude in microvolts (μV)	Norms	Remarkable range	Clinical implication probe
Alpha response			
Alpha(EC) – Alpha(EO)/Alpha(EO)	>50 %	<50 % or negative	If <50 % or negative, ask about traumatic stress (see also response at Cz), poor retention of information
			If 150 % +, ask about artistic interest or skills (visual arts, dance, poetry, carpentry, etc.)
Alpha recovery			
Alpha(EO) – Alpha(EO) after/ Alpha(EO)	<25 %	>25 %	If >25 %, ask about foggy thinking; ask about cognitive decline, sleep problems, medications
Theta(EO)/Beta(EO)	1.8–2.2	<1.8	If <1.8, ask about poor stress tolerance, racing thoughts, anxiety, inefficient self-quieting, sleep problems, symptoms of depression
		≪1.8	If ≪1.8, ask about predisposition to self-medicating behaviors (e.g., alcohol problem), GAD, and stress precipitated depression
		>3.0	If >3.0, ask about cognitive deficiencies or Asperger's patterns; also see F4/F3 Beta for symptoms. Also applies to T/B (EC), below
Theta(EC)/Beta(EC)	1.8–2.2	<1.5	If <1.5, ask about sleep disturbance. See Theta/Beta (EO), above, for description of probes
T/B (EO) – T/B (EC)/Min	> –25 %	< –25 %	If negative and < –25 %, question about sleep onset difficulties
			If % is positive, it indicates an increase from EO to EC
Total amplitude (EC)			
Theta(EC) + Alpha(EC) + Beta(EC)	<60	>60	If >60, ask about development delay, autistic spectrum behavior, marked cognitive deficits
Peak alpha frequency (EC)	>9.5	<9.5	If <9.5, ask about mental sluggishness
Peak alpha frequency (EO)	>9.5	<9.5	If <9.5, ask about mental sluggishness

Symptoms Associated with Remarkable Ranges at Positions F3 and F4

Interpretation of many of the remarkable ranges in the frontal lobes is rather straightforward, similar, in some respects, to interpretations at location Cz. One is looking for ratios among brainwave bandwidths that exceed clinical normative ranges. The more intriguing interpretations of frontal lobe activity, however, relate to the disparity or inequality of EEG activity between the frontal locations. The purpose of the ClinicalQ is to facilitate neurotherapy by demonstrating to the client that one really can determine the nature of their complaints simply by interpreting the limited brainwave data. One can be conventional about this process by letting the client describe their complaints and then showing the client where in the EEG one sees the "cause" of the problems. By far a more convincing and powerful demonstration of the efficacy of the ClinicalQ is to reverse this process and tell the client why he or she is sitting in your office. I routinely have clients, often with anger, tell me that I have told them more about their problems after 15 min, than they received after many hours of testing and follow-up sessions, often at a cost of many hundreds of dollars (see description of this process by Susan Olding in the Introduction to this book).

However, it is important to be organized and methodical in interpretation of the numerous combinations of markers identified by the ClinicalQ database. Considering only the various combinations of the two frontal locations for just three brainwave bands, the total number is well above 100. Further, when combined with the other sites in the ClinicalQ, the number becomes very large indeed. Because sites are correlated, we have expectations of what might be found at a location based on what was observed at a correlated site. For example, Common ADD (CADD) is related to an elevated Theta/Beta ratio over location Cz. When this is observed at Cz, it is also often found in the frontal regions (F3 and F4) as well. Hence, the remarkable finding, or comorbid condition, may be associated with frontal cortex patterns at variance with this expectation.

If the Theta/Beta ratio is above 2.20 in both areas, probe for cognitive deficiencies. One would usually find that the Theta/Beta ratio is also high at location Cz if it is high at F3 and F4 and that the deficiencies are similar to those associated with a high ratio at Cz. However, whenever the frontal lobes are inefficient, one may also find deficiencies associated with retrieval of information, impulse control, emotional volatility, and the like. For example, when the Theta/Beta ratio is elevated at both F3 and F4, there is a minor increase in ratings of behavioral perseveration ($t=2.00$, $p<0.05$, $df=426$). It is also interesting to note that individuals who rate themselves as very high on the "I fly off the handle" item have a Beta amplitude that, on average, is 12 % higher at both frontal locations relative to individuals who rate themselves as very low ($t=2.18$, $p=0.03$, $df=298$).

There are more specific frontal lobe signatures associated with the latter conditions, to be discussed shortly, but even without those specific brainwave patterns, some compromise of frontal lobe function may be apparent. This is particularly relevant with clients with traumatic brain injury. Whenever there is a head injury, regardless of the site of impact, the frontal lobes are usually implicated because of the way the brain sits in the cranial vault. Injury to the frontal regions is associated with mood volatility, anger problems, and impulse control issues.

If the Theta/Alpha ratio is below 1.00, probe for frontal Alpha ADD symptoms including problems with planning, organizing, sequencing, task completion, attention, and staying on task. Talkativeness is also often associated with this pattern. This is the form of ADD that we find is most frequently undiagnosed in young females. I assume that this is the case because a chatty, disorganized, flighty girl used to fit our stereotype of female behavior. I see many women in their 30s and 40s whose careers are a disaster and have had many unsuccessful relationships who show this high frontal Alpha form of ADD. They were not offered help as young students for, I presume, teachers (and perhaps parents) thought that these children were pleasant, sociable, and chatty but, alas, not intelligent. And unfortunately, they were treated in a manner consistent with this stereotype. The child, and then young woman, developed the belief that she had to struggle to keep up, and that, inevitably, she was not very bright. Her core emotional belief about herself became negative and disappointing and her life choices reflected that self-belief. These clients are usually depressed, angry, and disheartened and have to clear the emotional baggage as well as receive neurotherapy to correct the ADD. If the Theta/Alpha ratio is much below 1.00, one should also probe for pain disorders such as fibromyalgia, chronic fatigue, and sleep disturbance.

Note that the Theta/Alpha ratio can be low either because Alpha is high or Theta is low in amplitude. High frontal Alpha is associated with Alpha being elevated not Theta being deficient. Theta deficiency is associated with poor stress tolerance, anxiety, and hypervigilance whereas elevated Alpha amplitude is the ADD condition associated with problems with planning, organizing, sequencing, and following through on tasks.

In a group of 24 children drawn from our database with Theta/Alpha ratios below 1.10, 16.7 % were rated, by a parent, as not having an attention problem whereas 50.0 % were rated as having a serious attention problem ($z=2.78$, $p<0.01$, $N=24$).

For a sample of 118 adults with a Theta/Alpha ratio below 0.85, the number reporting a serious problem with concentration (rating of 4 or 5 on the 5-point scale) was 55.1 % as opposed to 14.4 % who rated that they had no or a minimal problem. This difference was significant ($z=7.27$, $p<0.001$, $N=118$). For a sample of adults with a Theta/Alpha ratio below 1.10, 22.5 % reported their concentration problem as severe (rating of 5) whereas 4.2 % rated themselves as having no (rating of 1) problem with concentration ($z=5.54$, $p<0.001$, $N=191$).

High frontal Alpha amplitude is also related to client complaints of emotional dysregulation. As will be discussed in the following chapter, clients diagnosed with a "bipolar" disorder are very likely to have elevated frontal Alpha amplitude. On the other hand, clients with trauma markers and those who report that they are easily frightened have, on average, deficient Alpha amplitude in the frontal regions. Clients whose Alpha amplitude was at least 2.3 times less than Theta Amplitude were 44.1 % more likely to rate themselves as "very anxious" as compared with those whose Theta amplitude was less than 1.8 times that of the Alpha amplitude (i.e., those whose Theta and Alpha amplitudes were consistent with the frequency inversely related to amplitude algorithm) ($z=2.18$, $p<0.03$, $N=658$) (Table 2.4).

Table 2.4 Basic clinical probes for locations F3 and/or F4

Formula Amplitude in microvolts (μV)	Norms	Remarkable range	Clinical implication probe
Theta(EC)/Beta(EC)	<2.2	>2.2	If >2.2, ask about cognitive deficiencies associated with retrieval of information, impulse control, emotional volatility, etc. Ask about depression in adults and impulse control in children
Theta(EC)/Alpha(EC) (*Note*: Verify that low ratio is excessive Alpha amplitude not deficient Theta amplitude)	1.2–1.6	<1.0	If <1.0, ask about frontal Alpha ADD—problems with organization, sequencing, sustained focus, planning, task completion, staying on task, talkativeness
		≪0.8	If ≪0.8, ask about fibromyalgia, chronic fatigue, and sleep disturbance
Total amplitude (EC)			
Theta(EC) + Alpha(EC) + Beta(EC)	<60	>60	If >60, ask about development delays, autism spectrum disorder (especially if O1 Theta is high and the anterior cingulate gyrus is "hot"); memory/cognitive deficits in adults

Symptoms Associated with Disparities Between Locations F3 and F4

Disparities in the form of imbalances in the frontal lobes are a rich source of information about the client. Henriques and Davidson (1990) have reported that there is a relationship between imbalances in frontal Alpha and depression. Individuals with depression were more likely to have left dominant Alpha, and several studies have indicated improved mood states with reductions in left frontal Alpha amplitude.

Activation of the frontal lobes can be associated with several neurological indicators including the left frontal Alpha dominance, cited above, but also greater Beta amplitude on the right relative to the left, greater Theta in the left relative to the right, and greater Theta/Beta ratio in left relative to the right. From our database, clients were selected who rated themselves as having no depression (1 on a 5-point scale), and those clients who designated on the intake form that depression was the reason they were seeking treatment.

Of the clients who self-designated depression, 89.2 % showed one or more of the above frontal indicators (i.e., 15 % or greater Alpha or Theta amplitude in the left relative to the right frontal cortex, greater Beta amplitude in the right relative to the left, or greater Theta/Beta ratio in the left relative to the right). Of the clients who rated themselves as a 4 or 5 (out of 5) on depression, 51.9 % had the Beta marker, 44.6 % had the Alpha marker, 34.4 % had the Theta marker, and 33.3 % had the Theta/Beta marker. Those clients with no depression markers rated themselves about equally (32 % to 34 %) as 1–2, 3, or 4–5 on the 5-point depression scale. For clients rating themselves high on the depression scale (4 or 5), the significance of the difference in proportions between those with no depression markers and those with the Beta marker was $p<0.001$ ($z=7.67$, $N=704$); between those with no markers and the Alpha marker was $p<0.001$ ($z=4.03$, $N=597$); between those with no markers and those with one or more depression markers was $p<0.0001$ ($z=16.78$, $N=742$). Of the clients rating themselves as 4 or 5 on the depression scale with no depression markers, 86.1 % had a deficiency in the Theta/Beta ratio (<1.6) at location O1 ($z=17.96$, $p<0.001$, $N=135$). It appears as though clients with anxiety markers, with no depression markers, may be defining their anxious state/symptoms as depression rather than sequellae of anxiety. Later in this book several cases of anxiety-based "depression" are examined. These cases often reveal problem of long history of unsuccessful treatment of depression when the putative cause had been untreated.

When interpreting the meaningfulness of frontal imbalances, it is important to consider some markers that indicate shadow or correlated symptoms. The clinician should be mindful that the 15 % threshold for the principal depression marker (Beta marker) is only a guide for directing clinical probes during the intake session. One obviously does not ignore the Beta imbalance if it is 14.5, so it is important to consider the shadow markers when forming hypotheses about the clinical condition. When the Beta amplitude is over 15 % greater on the right relative to the left, 51.9 % of clients rate themselves as highly depressed. When the imbalance is between 4 % and 8 %, 25.5 % rate themselves high on depression, but when the imbalance is between 8 % and 15 %, 39.3 % do so. All of these comparisons are statistically significant ($p<0.001$).

The Beta marker is also related to other symptoms as rated by clients. Those rating themselves as easily irritated have on average 7.5 % greater amplitude in the right ($t=2.03$, $p<0.001$, $df=452$) and those "easily frightened" 12.8 % higher ($t=2.62$, $p<0.001$, $df=403$). Those clients rating themselves as high on "I have sleep problems" had, on average, a F4 > F3 Beta amplitude ratio that was 248.6 % greater in the right frontal cortex relative to those rating themselves as a one on the five-point scale ($t=3.79$, $p<0.001$, $df=465$). Further, the Beta amplitude in the right for those rating themselves as high on the sleep problems item was, on average, 10.5 % higher than for those clients rating themselves as without sleep problems ($t=2.08$, $p<0.04$, $df=465$).

It is useful to note that many clients who come for treatment may not be aware of their depressed mood state. Often clients will define their condition as anxiety, poor motivation, poor energy, lack of interest, and the like, rather than the more fundamental condition associated with these conditions, which is depression.

Elevated Beta amplitude in the right frontal cortex, relative to the left, is associated with predisposition to depressed mood states. Clients who rate themselves high on depression have a Beta amplitude at both frontal locations that is, on average, 10.6 % greater than those who rate themselves as not having depression ($t=1.93$, $p<0.05$, $df=440$). The self-rated depressed clients have, on average, Beta amplitude 12.8 % greater in the right relative to the left frontal cortex ($t=3.31$, $p<0.001$, $df=734$). Based on right to left percentage ratio difference, the amplitude percentage is 103.2 % greater in the right relative to the left ($t=2.19$, $p<0.03$, $df=366$).

In addition to depression, high activation of the right frontal cortex as indicated by high amplitude Alpha in the left frontal cortex is related to significantly lower levels of natural killer cell activity (Kang et al. 1991). Further, in this study the group with the high right frontal cortex activation also had higher IgM levels indicating the possibility of recent subclinical viral infection. In my experience, clients showing these EEG patterns routinely complain of cognitive inefficiencies and often report having recently experienced a cold, a flu-like reaction, or increased allergy reactions.

When F4 Beta is more than 15 % greater than F3 Beta or F3 Theta/Beta is more than 15 % greater than F4, probe for predisposition to depressed mood states. In young children, this may manifest not as frank sadness but rather as disinterest, lethargy, and poor motivation for any activities other than isolating activities such as TV or video games.

When F4 Theta is more than 15 % greater than F3 Theta or F3 Theta/Beta ratio is 20 % less than F4 probe for emotional volatility, anger management problems, and emotional impulse control. Sometimes in adults, particularly males, one finds emotional restriction (i.e., very narrow emotional window) that seems to be a response to, or effort to control, emotional volatility.

From the client database, clients with F4 Theta amplitude that was at least 10 % greater than F3 Theta amplitude and a second group where the Theta amplitude was less than 5 % greater were selected. From that group those who indicated on the intake questionnaire that they were easily irritated or annoyed were categorized on the basis of the above disparities in frontal lobe Theta. Significant differences were found only for the female clients. Of those who rated themselves high on the easily irritated questionnaire item, 58.0 % had 10 % or greater Theta amplitude in the right frontal cortex as compared with the left whereas 34.0 % had disparities less than 5 % ($z=2.48$, $p<0.02$, $N=50$).

Males were more willing to admit to a positive emotion in that 45.3 % of those with 10 % or greater Theta amplitude in the right frontal cortex relative to the left rated themselves high on the “laugh a lot” questionnaire item as compared to 26.4 % with imbalance ratios less than 5 % ($z=3.11$, $p<0.001$, $N=28$). For females, 62.5 % of those with Theta amplitude imbalances greater than 10 % rated themselves high on the “laugh a lot” item as compared to 20.0 % with imbalances less than 5 % ($z=5.31$, $p<0.001$, $N=53$). Overall, without regard to gender, clients with Theta amplitude 20 % higher in the right relative to those with imbalance below 10 % rated themselves 12.8 % higher on the “Easily frightened” item ($t=3.00$, $p<0.003$, $df=407$).

The proportion of clients with Theta/Beta ratios 20 % or stronger on the right, compared with those with ratios between 0 and 10 %, rating themselves as high (4 or 5 on the 5-point scale): 27.2 % more (0.54 vs. 0.42) on “I am very anxious” ($z=2.01$, $p<0.05$, $df=329$); 59.2 % more (0.33 vs. 0.21) on “Easily frightened” ($z=2.46$, $p<0.02$, $df=326$); 22.9 % more (0.53 vs. 0.43) on “Too willing to please others” ($z=1.98$, $p<0.05$, $N=407$); 54.8 % more (0.27 vs 0.18) on “Easily frightened” ($z=2.34$, $p<0.02$, $N=405$).

As discussed above, when Alpha amplitude is greater in the left, clients are more likely to rate themselves as “Depressed.” Like Alpha, when Theta amplitude is elevated in the left relative to the right frontal cortex then the right side is more active than the left, the hallmark for predisposition to depressed mood states. Comparing clients with Theta amplitude between 0 and 10 % greater in the right versus those clients with Theta amplitude more than 15 % greater in the left, the proportion of the latter rating themselves high on depression is 50 % greater than the contrast group of clients (0.46 vs. 0.31; $z=2.14$, $p=0.03$, $N=271$). Similarly, when the Theta/Beta ratio is greater on the left relative to the right frontal cortex, then the right is more active than the left, again the hallmark for predisposition to depressed mood states. Comparing clients with Theta/Beta ratio between 0 and 10 % greater in the left versus those clients with Theta/Beta ratio more than 15 % greater in the left, the proportion of the latter rating themselves high on depression is 32.9 % greater than the contrast group of clients (0.42 vs. 0.32; $z=2.00$, $p=0.05$, $N=346$).

When F4 Alpha is greater than F3 Alpha, probe for oppositional, defiant, and socially aggressive or socially indifferent behavior. Of 59 children drawn from our client base who had an Alpha amplitude imbalance of 10 % or greater, right relative to left, 32.2 % were rated by a parent as “easy to anger”. Of this same group with the 10 % disparity, only 3.4 % were rated as low (1 on a 5-point scale) on the “easy to anger” question. This difference is statistically significant ($z=4.43$, $p<0.001$, $N=59$). Similarly, from this same sample of 59 children, 3.4 % were rated by a parent as not defiant as compared with 28.8 % who were rated as strongly defiant ($z=4.03$, $p<0.001$, $N=59$).

If Total Amplitude is considerably greater than the clinical normative range of below 60, probe for developmental delays, autism spectrum behaviors (particularly if O1 Theta is high and the anterior cingulate gyrus is "hot"), and memory and cognitive deficits in adults.

Probe for fibromyalgia, chronic fatigue, and viral infections when F4 Beta is more than 15 % greater than F3, and F4 Theta is more than 15 % greater than F3, and/or F4 Theta/Alpha is greater than 15 % less than F3, particularly when O1 Theta/Beta ratio is less than 1.50. Dr. Stuart Donaldson (1998) found that clients reporting a diagnosis of fibromyalgia often showed slow frequency dominance in the frontal regions. Clients rating themselves high on fatigue had, on average, 11.9 % higher Theta amplitude in the right relative to clients rating themselves as a 1 ($t=2.46$, $p<0.02$, $df=476$; Clients rating themselves as high on fatigue also had, on average, 10.2 % greater right, relative to left, Theta amplitude ($t=2.18$, $p<0.03$, $df=476$) and those rating themselves as easily irritated averaged 7.6 % greater right Theta amplitude ($t=2.26$, $p<0.03$, $df=606$). Clients rating themselves as "physically unwell" had, on average, 9 % higher Theta amplitude in the right relative to those clients rating themselves a 1 on this dimension ($t=2.22$, $p<0.03$, $df=438$).

In my experience with fibromyalgia clients, although the dominant frequency is often in the Alpha or Theta range, high amplitude slow frequency brainwave activity is found more frequently on the right relative to the left frontal regions. Further, in my experience, these individuals also show deficiencies in the Theta/Beta ratio in the occipital region and show the Beta frontal imbalance form of depression, in addition to the right dominant slow frequency amplitude. In a sample of 30 female clients, those with self-reported previous diagnosis of fibromyalgia and matched contrast clients of the same age, the former were more likely to have greater Theta, Alpha, and Beta amplitude on the right relative to the left. For the fibromyalgia group, 71.4 % had a disparity of at least 10 % for all three brainwave bands as opposed to 30.4 % for the matched contrast group ($z=4.56$, $p<0.01$, $N=30$).

It is also interesting to note that slowing in the frontal regions, again in my experience more frequently in the right relative to the left, is associated with viral infections, toxicity, and allergic reactions. Westmoreland (1993) and Ochs (cited in Donaldson 1998) report that these conditions are often associated with increased slow wave amplitude in the frontal regions. In my experience, when I find that a client, such as an ADD child, shows a regression of behavior and a correlated increase in Theta amplitude, the cause is often that the child has experienced a cold or flu or is having an exacerbation of an allergic condition. It is interesting that this increased slow frequency can be reduced with neurotherapy and the related conditions improved.

A sample of 15 clients was drawn from the clinical database who had an imbalance in Beta amplitude with the left being more than 13 % greater than the right. This group had no other frontal lobe imbalances that exceeded the clinical thresholds. Of that group, 100 % rated themselves at three or greater on a five-point scale "I am very anxious," and 71.4 % rated themselves at four or greater. I now include a probe for anxiety if I find this imbalance in Beta amplitude between the frontal lobes.

We are in the process of looking at the fluctuations in the imbalances in frontal Beta amplitude over time for clients diagnosed with bipolar disorder. It may be that the mechanism associated with the flip/flopping between manic and depressive episodes is associated with corresponding imbalances in the frontal regions; depression when the Beta amplitude is dominant in the right, and manic when the Beta amplitude is dominant in the left. I also usually find that Alpha amplitude is elevated in both frontal regions with bipolar clients, which is associated with high frontal Alpha ADD symptoms. Hence, the Beta imbalances may be associated with the valance whereas the general elevated Alpha is associated with the emotional dysregulation.

The experienced intuitive clinician will find frontal lobe brainwave patterning a very fertile arena for discovering unique but consistent patterns associated with various unique behaviors (Table 2.5).

Symptoms Associated with Remarkable Patterns at Location Fz

One of the most exciting discoveries was that the activity of the Anterior Cingulate Gyrus (ACG) could be assessed from location Fz by measuring HiBeta, Beta, and Gamma (Swingle 2002, February). In addition to providing neurological evidence for certain behaviors, this discovery also introduced the exciting possibility of treating symptoms associated with this subcortical structure neurotherapeutically with surface electrodes.

When I was at McLean Hospital, a neurosurgeon asked me to collaborate on a study of the effects of cingulotomy on the Autonomic Nervous System (ANS). Cingulotomy is a last resort treatment for intractable obsessive–compulsive behaviors and he presumed that the mechanism of beneficial change implicated the ANS. Several studies of the long-term effects of cingulotomy (e.g., Dougherty et al. 2002; Kim et al. 2003) indicate that only 25–35 % of patients receive symptom relief from this radical irreversible treatment, so it is indeed exciting that neurotherapy can access the ACG. We now have several neurotherapeutic protocols that effect change directly in the ACG that has proved very efficient and effective in the treatment of disorders associated with this structure.

For the ClinicalQ assessment, an eyes-closed sample is obtained of Delta (2 Hz), HiBeta-Gamma (28–40 Hz), and Beta (16–25 Hz). One must be particularly careful about artifact contamination of Delta. I usually take 5 epochs of 8 or fewer seconds and select the epoch(s) where I see no physical movement of the client, paying particular attention to facial and eye movements.

If Delta is above 9 μV, probe for cognitive deficits. Higher values can be associated with a number of conditions such as developmental delays and pain. Usually, one will see some remarkable patterns in the data obtained at F3 and F4 when Delta is also high. In such cases, I rely more heavily on the F3 and F4 data for interpreting the client's complaints.

Table 2.5 Basic clinical probes for imbalances between locations F3 and F4

Formula Amplitude in microvolts (μV)	Norms	Remarkable range	Clinical implication probe
[T/B (F3) – T/B (F4)]/Min	+<20 %	–>20 %	If negative and >20 %, ask about emotional volatility, anger management problems, emotional impulse control. In males, in particular, emotional restrictions (very narrow emotional window) that seem to be a response to or effort to control emotional volatility
T(F3) – T(F4)/Min	<10 %	F4 > 15 %	If F4 Theta > 15 % to F3 Theta, ask about emotional volatility or conversely restricted emotional range
		F3 > 15 %	If F3 Theta > 15 % to F4 Theta, ask about depression in adults and impulse control in children
A(F3) – A(F4)/Min	<10 %	F3 > 15 %	If F3 Alpha > 15 % to F4 Alpha, ask about depression in adults and impulse control in children
		F4 > 15 %	If F4 Alpha > 15 % to F3 Alpha, ask about oppositional, defiant and socially aggressive or socially indifferent behavior; general elevated Alpha associated with emotional dysregulation
B(F3) – B(F4)/Min	<10 %	F4 > 15 %	If F4 Beta > 15 % to F3 Beta, ask about predisposition to depressed mood states in adults and impulse control in children
		F4 > 20 %	If F4 Beta > 20 % to F3 Beta and F4/F3 (Theta) > 20 % and F4 T/A > –20 % < F3 T/A (particularly when O1 T/B < 1.5), ask about fibromyalgia and chronic fatigue
		F3>15 %	If F3 Beta>15% to F4 Beta, ask about anxiety, poor stress tolerance

Elevated Delta and Theta amplitude in the frontal regions is also often associated with the cognitive deficiencies following Lyme's disease and with clients with Systemic Lupus Erythematous (SLE) (Chabot and Sigal 1995; Ritchlin et al. 1992). SLE can manifest in many ways, affecting many different organs and areas of the body. For cognitive deficiencies, suppressing the slow frequency amplitude in the frontal regions of the brain can be very effective. For other complications of SLE, often, peripheral biofeedback is the treatment of choice. For example, a SLE client that I treated (Swingle 1992, pp. 117–120) had major circulation deficiencies in his legs. This condition was very successfully treated with thermal biofeedback of the feet combined with hypnosis and some relaxation exercises. This client had been told that he was at risk of requiring amputation of his right foot and, when I first saw him, he was on 60 mg of prednisone per day. Follow-up at 20 months posttreatment indicated that the client was pain-free, the circulation in his right foot continued to be adequate, and his prednisone level averaged about 2 mg/day. He reported that when he experienced bouts of severe stress, he would often markedly increase his home relaxation program, and his physician would increase his prednisone level for a short period.

Clients with a history of Lyme's disease often have EEG patterns similar to those frequently found in clients with fibromyalgia. A 50-year-old female client with Lyme's disease, for example, had a Theta/Beta ratio of 1.18 at O1. The elevated slow frequency amplitude in the frontal regions, however, is often more pronounced in the right relative to the left. In this case, for example, the Theta/Beta ratio at location F4 was 4.44 whereas on the left (F3) it was 2.62. Alpha amplitude, likewise, was elevated in the right (29 % higher) relative to the left. This client also showed the trauma profile as well, in that there was no Alpha response at either location O1 or Cz.

A woman of similar age with a diagnosis of fibromyalgia and chronic fatigue likewise had a deficient Theta/Beta ratio at location O1 (1.17) and deficient Alpha response at O1 and Cz (17.0 % and 16.4 %, respectively). Her Theta/Beta ratio in the right (F4) was 29.8 % greater than in the left (F3). Although elevated Delta is also commonly associated with these conditions, in the above two illustrative cases, the Delta amplitude was only modestly elevated (about 11 % on average). Hence, the cognitive deficiencies experienced by the above two clients were reflected in the elevated Theta and Alpha in the frontal regions and less so in the Delta amplitude.

When the ratio of 28–40Hz/16–25Hz amplitudes is less than 0.45 probe for excessive passiveness. When the ratio is above 0.55 probe for stubborn, obsessive, compulsive, and perseverative behavior patterns. For example, in a group of 168 clients from our database with ratios above 0.60 or below 0.40, 51.5 % of those with the higher ratio rated themselves as anxious whereas 39.0 % of those with a ratio below 0.40 rated themselves as anxious (4 or 5 on a 5-point scale). This difference is statistically significant ($z=2.36$, $p<0.03$, $N=168$). Similarly, 28 % of the clients with the higher ratio rated themselves as needing to "check things I know I have already done" (4 or 5 on a 5-point scale) as compared with 10 % of those clients with ratios 0.40 or below ($z=3.66$, $p<0.002$, $N=167$).

Compared with clients with ratios in the normative range (0.45 to 0.55), those with ratios below 0.40 rated themselves, on average, 38.8 % higher on "Too willing to please others" ($t=2.35$, $p<0.02$, $df=298$). Forty six percent of those with ratios in the normative range rated themselves high on "Too willing to please other" whereas 64 % of those with ratios below 0.40 rated themselves as high on this dimension ($z=2.35$, $p<0.02$, $N=300$).

In a sample of 79 children seen in our clinic for various complaints, those with a ratio below 0.40 were half (19 %) as likely to be rated by a parent as "stubborn" as compared with those (40 %) with ratios above 0.60 ($z=2.86$, $p<0.005$, $N=79$). Children with the lower ratios were also less likely to be rated by a parent as "obsessive" (25 % vs. 9 %, $z=2.60$, $p<0.009$, $N=76$). Ratios above 0.55 are common in autistic spectrum behaviors, and one should assume a "hot midline" when treating autistic spectrum disordered clients who show this pattern.

One is extremely cautious about stimulation protocols over the midline when the midline is "hot" to avoid the possibility of seriously exacerbating autistic behavior. The magnitude of the departure from the normative range of 0.45–0.55 guides the nature of the probes. At 0.60, for example, I would suggest that the client is stubborn and may find it difficult to get troubling thoughts out of mind. At a ratio above 0.80, I would probe more obsessive/compulsive themes in behavior. A ratio of 0.45 would suggest that the person is open minded and conciliatory, whereas at 0.35 I would probe for more problematic passivity.

We have been consulting for marriage and family therapists who have couples who appear treatment resistant. Our assessment is principally focused on the ACG of both individuals. If the ACG is "hot" in both individuals, then the only counseling strategy that seems effective is the "stop" procedure of an agreement between the parties that either can hold up a hand to stop communication at any point. The presumption is that after a cooling down period, the couple can resume the argument toward resolution of the disagreement.

If the ACG is hot in one person and underactive in the other, we often find the pattern of dominance and control to the point of explosive outbursts from the more passive person. There are other patterns associated with other inefficient interpersonal interactions. Our approach is to normalize the ACG in both individuals and then resume the couple counseling.

Thompson (2006) have a similar measure of activity presumed to reflect the activity of the ACG. Their ratio is the amplitude of 26–34 Hz/13–15 Hz. The Thompsons suggest that a ratio over 1.50 is indicative of a "busy brain" associated with interference with attention and focus, anxiety conditions, and perseverative behavior and thought patterns. These data were analyzed using the LORETA program, and it was determined that, indeed, the origin of this high frequency Beta activity was the anterior cingulate (Brodmann Area 24). Hammond (2005) also reports that clients with obsessive–compulsive disorder often have excessive high frequency amplitude over this region.

The second datum that is obtained from the ACG assessment is the sum of the amplitudes of 28–40 Hz and 16–25 Hz. If that sum is greater than 15, probe for fretting and worrying behaviors and assume a hot midline in the treatment of autistic spectrum behaviors. In addition, if the sum of the above is high, one must be cautious in interpreting the ratio of the two amplitudes. Extremely high Beta amplitude, for example, may result in a minimal ratio that is not indicative of passive behavior.

In a sample of 98 clients taken from our database, of those with a sum of the amplitude of 28–40 Hz plus 16–25 Hz greater than 18, 9.5 % rated themselves low (1 or 2, out of 5) in anxiety whereas those with sums 12 or less, 28.6 % rated themselves low in anxiety ($z=3.54$, $p<0.003$, $N=98$). Similarly, those in the low sum group rated themselves as less troubled with annoying thoughts (38.2 %) as compared with the high sum group (19.0 %)($z=3.20$, $p<0.003$, $N=97$). Clients rating themselves high on depression also show, on average, a 15 % higher sum ($t=2.51$, $p<0.02$, $df=368$) and those saying "they do not have much to look forward to" have 10 % higher sum ($t=2.57$, $p<0.02$, $df=449$). An 11.2 % elevated sum is also found with clients who rate themselves as "physically unwell" ($t=2.82$, $p=0.005$, $df=438$). And as might be expected, those who report sleep problems have a sum that is 12 % greater than those not reporting sleep problems ($t=2.50$, $p<0.02$, $df=465$).

Clients with markers for elevated activity in this region, as indicated above, tend to rate themselves higher on items associated with perseverative thought processes. The ratings of having annoying or disturbing thoughts also correlates with other self-ratings indicating potential negative emotional effects of this elevated neurological activity. The self-ratings of not being able to "…get rid annoying or disturbing thoughts" correlates with: "…too willing to please…" ($r=0.30$); "easily frightened" ($r=0.43$), "unwell" ($r=0.25$); "depressed" ($r=0.42$); "anxious" ($r=0.47$); "not much to look forward to" ($r=0.34$); poor "concentration" ($r=0.31$); and irritability ($r=0.37$). All correlations are $N=914$, $p<0.001$.

The second assessment at location Fz is the ratio of slow Alpha (or Lo-Alpha) to fast Alpha (or Hi-Alpha). Other systems may assess the dominant (Peak) Frequency (PF) of the Alpha band activity, but in the ClinicalQ we assess the ratio of the amplitude of 8–9Hz/11–12Hz. The historical reason for this measurement is that it is available with any EEG platform and provides an efficient metric for use with brain-driving protocols, to be reviewed later in this book. The Lo/Hi Alpha ratio correlates with Alpha PF ($r=0.81$, $p<0.0001$, $df=101$). In general, the lower this ratio the better. Low ratios reflect more efficient brain functioning. If the ratio is above 1.50, probe for age related memory declines, developmental delays, cognitive deficits, and sleep disorders. It is interesting to note that clients rating themselves high on depression have a Lo/Hi Alpha ratio that is, on average, 12.5 % lower than those rating themselves as not being depressed. This is consistent with research on veterans with PTSD who also show faster Alpha Peak Frequency which may be associated with elevated vigilance. Clients rating themselves as have difficulty with behavioral regulation (doing things because they cannot resist) also show a lower ratio, on average of about 11 % ($t=2.25$, $p<0.03$, $df=425$).

A sample of 126 adults with Alpha amplitude ratios above 2.00 or below 1.00 were compared on the self-rating of often feeling tired. Almost twice as many adults with the low ratio rated themselves low (1 out of 5) on this dimension (30 %) as did those clients with the high ratios (15.2 %) ($z=3.36$, $p<0.001$, $N=126$).

Also clients with the higher ratios were more likely to rate themselves as having problems with concentration and forgetfulness (55.3 %) as compared to those with the lower ratios (47.9 %) ($z=1.85$, $p<0.06$, $N=126$).

Slowing of Alpha has also been reported in clients with Chronic Fatigue Syndrome (CFS) consistent with the hypothesis that CFS is caused by a viral infection (Schwartz et al. 1994). Alpha Peak Frequency is also related to reported physical unwellness; clients rating themselves low on this dimension had APF that was, on average, 7 % faster than those rating themselves high on the "physically unwell" question ($t=2.02$, $p<0.05$, $df=55$). High Alpha is also associated with cognitive performance, and increasing high Alpha with neurofeedback enhances cognitive performance (Hanslmayr et al. 2005). Clients with brain injury have slower APF relative to healthy controls and short-term memory is also positively correlated with peak Alpha frequency (Angelakis 2003). In addition, the larger the decrease in high Alpha under task conditions, the lower the intelligence of the subject (Doppelmayr and Klimesch 2003). Relaxation exercises (e.g., meditation) can reduce APF (Cahn and Polich 2006), and cognitive preparedness is associated with increased APF. A study of veterans with PTSD found elevated APF which suggests that APF may be associated with hypervigilance (Wahbeh and Oken 2013).

In general, faster APF is associated with better performance on cognitive tasks, memory, and has been found to improve response to a wide variety of medications and treatments. A drop in APF is generally associated with a drop in performance (Klimesch et al. 1993). Task activity increases APF but only in the hemisphere dominant for the specific task (Osaka 1984). See the section on neurotherapy in general medical practice for more details on the relationship of APF to brain efficiency.

For the ClinicalQ assessment, an eyes-closed sample of Delta (2 Hz) amplitude is obtained. When Delta amplitude is high, ask about problems with concentration, forgetfulness, and comprehension. In a sample of 92 clients taken from our adult database, for example, more than twice as many clients (30 %) indicated that they had no problem with concentration when their Delta amplitude was below 5 μV than clients whose Delta amplitude was above 10 μV (14 %) ($z=2.31$, $p=0.01$, $N=92$). Of 53 clients from our database who rated themselves as either a 1 (no problem with concentration) or 5 (major problem with concentration), 20 % of the former had Delta amplitudes above 8 μV, whereas 54 % of the latter had ratios above 8 ($z=4.93$, $p<0.001$, $N=53$). Comparing clients with Delta amplitude below 7 with those above 12, 33 % more of the latter rated themselves high on "hard to concentrate" ($z=2.32$, $p<0.02$, $df=453$).

Clients who rate themselves high on depression have, on average, 15 % greater Delta amplitude compared with clients rating themselves at level one ($t=2.06$, $p<0.04$, $df=340$). Those clients rating themselves high on fatigue also have 15 % greater Delta amplitude, on average ($t=2.30$, $p<0.03$, $df=446$), and 12.6 % greater Delta if they rate themselves as physically unwell ($t=2.50$. $p<0.02$, $df=406$).

When assessing seriously demoralized children who have come to the conclusion that they are stupid because of attention deficiencies, a low ratio of Lo-Alpha to Hi-Alpha amplitude provides another opportunity to encourage feelings of self-worth and optimism. The power of these positive interpretative interventions cannot be overestimated. In one recent situation, a little girl had a ratio of 0.98 and I elaborated at length about the significance of this "great" ratio concluding with the statement that she had the brain of a "rocket scientist." The child's mother called me stating that the change in her daughter's behavior was "unbelievable." The child reported to her family, "Dr. Swingle said I have the brain of a rocket scientist" and her attitude toward homework and school was completely changed. Her teacher, who called the mother to comment on this remarkable shift in attitude, echoed this change (Table 2.6).

Discussion

Recognizing the enormous number of profiles that can be generated from the five-point assessment, considering only a few brainwave bandwidths, let us try to summarize some of the more prominent patterns one is likely to encounter in clinical practice. The basic ClinicalQ probes are detailed on the summary charts included in this chapter as well as in Appendix A. Although the basic probes are itemized in the summary charts, careful consideration of the ClinicalQ data can provide the clinician with a very detailed and accurate qualitative assessment of the client's clinical state. The precision of the ClinicalQ provides the clinician with important insight into the client's condition and, without any information from the client, provides the clinician with the ability to show the client how the information from the brain allows the clinician to understand the client's condition without any prior information but much more importantly to be able to identify the areas in the brain to focus treatment to improve the client's condition.

Again, this can be addressed in two ways, top-down or bottom-up. If a client presents with the compliant of "fibromyalgia" as diagnosed by the referring physician, what should be the expected ClinicalQ profile? As suggested by the data presented above, the clinician might expect a Theta/Beta deficiency at location O1, a trauma marker at O1 and/or Cz, a depression marker in the frontal cortex, and the right frontal slow frequency excess identified by Dr. Stu Donaldson. Far more impressive to the client, however, is to reverse the process and ask the client, based on the ClinicalQ data, if they experience sleep problems, poor stress tolerance, chatter in the brain, depressed mood states, and fibromyalgia and/or chronic fatigue.

This is not a "party trick." The ClinicalQ is a very important clinical intervention. The ClinicalQ is the basis for the initial psychotherapy session with the client. It strongly focuses the client on the therapeutic metaphor that their problem(s) are reflected in brain activity, that their complaint(s) are validated, and that the clinician knows precisely where to go to treat the condition and what other complementary therapies will be helpful to maximize therapeutic benefit. With this in mind, the primary indicators at the five ClinicalQ locations are reviewed. Further refinements and subtleties regarding the qualitative features of the client's cognitive/emotional/physical condition are indicated by the data presented previously as will become apparent as the clinician gains experience with the ClinicalQ procedure.

Table 2.6 Basic clinical probes for locations Fz

Fz Amplitude in microvolts (μV)	Norms	Remarkable range	Clinical implication probe
Delta (EC)	<9.0	>9.0	If >9.0, ask about cognitive deficits such as problems with concentration, forgetfulness and comprehension
			Higher values can be associated with developmental delays and pain; will usually see remarkable patterns in F3 and F4 if Delta is high
HiBetaGamma/Beta (EC)	0.45–0.55	<0.45	If <0.45, ask about passiveness
		>0.55	If >0.55, ask about stubborn behavior, OC tendencies or OCD, perseveration in autistic spectrum behaviors. Assume hot midline (anterior cingulate gyrus) in treatment of autistic spectrum behaviors
		>0.60 <0.40	If >0.60 or <0.40, ask about anxiety
		>0.80	If >0.80, ask about O/C behaviors
		<0.35	If <0.35, problematic passivity
			Caution! If there is extremely elevated Beta, minimal ratio may result that does not indicate passive behavior
Sum HiBetaGamma + Beta	<15	>15	If >15, ask about autistic spectrum behavior. Implications of elevated HiBetaGamma/Beta described above apply only if sum of amplitudes of HiBeta + Beta < 15
			If >15, but HiBeta/Beta is within normative range, ask about fretting and assume hot midline in treatment of autistic spectrum behaviors
		<15	When <15, clients reported less annoying thoughts
		>16	If >16, "hot" midline
LoAlpha(EC)/HiAlpha(EC)	1.0–1.5	>1.5	If >1.5, ask about cognitive inefficiency, age-related deficits in memory and cognitive processing, and sleep
			If >1.5, ask about problems with concentration and forgetfulness
		≫1.5	If ≫1.5, ask about developmental delays, marked cognitive deficits
			The lower this ratio, the better, as it reflects more efficient brain functioning
Peak Frequency Alpha (EC)	>9.5	<9.5	If <9.5 ask about mental sluggishness

At location Cz: When the Theta/Beta ratio is above about 2.2, a bit higher for very young children, probe for problems with attention, focus, and retrieval of information. If the Alpha response is below 30 %, or seems blunted when observing the raw signal, probe for exposure to severe emotional stress. If the Alpha return is slow, above about 25 %, probe for problems with retention and retrieval of information. If the Theta/Beta ratio increases substantially under cognitive challenge, when the client is reading or counting backwards, probe again for the characteristics associated with attention problems. If the Theta/SMR ratio is above about three, probe for involuntary movement concerns including tics and seizure disorders. If the total amplitude at that location is above about 60 μV, probe for cognitive delays and problems with attention, focus, and retrieval of information. If one finds excesses in slow frequency amplitude over the sensory motor cortex (Cz), then one should also expect to find elevations in the Theta/Beta ratio in the frontal cortex as well. The correlations between the Theta/Beta ratio at Cz and the frontal regions F3 and F4 are in the range of 0.60 and at Fz the coefficient is 0.46.

At location O1: It is important to recall that Dr. Peniston had remarkable results from increasing the Theta amplitude at location O1 with chronic hospitalized alcoholics. On the other hand, it is also important to recall that senior executives, Olympic level athletes, and accomplished artists often have markedly low Theta/Beta ratios at this location. However, the latter are seeking optimizing of performance whereas the former are seeking relief from clinical complaints. Focusing exclusively on clinical clients, deficiency in the Theta/Beta ratio at O1 is associated with problems with "turning the brain off," poor sleep, poor stress tolerance, feelings of anxiety, problems with concentration, and focus. Clients in poor physical health often have marked deficiencies in the Theta/Beta ratio in this region. A most important implication of the low Theta/Beta ratio at 01 is a predisposition for self-medicating behavior. Self-medication can include: alcohol abuse, prescription medication abuse, street drugs, gambling, Internet addiction, sex addiction, among others.

At locations F3 and F4: The experienced clinician will find the frontal cortex a treasure trove of information for defining the qualitative profile of the client both cognitively and emotionally. This is where the ClinicalQ is most productive for it identifies the often subtle neurological influences on the client's cognitive/emotional state.

The first item to consider is if the spectral array of the brainwave activity for the two locations satisfies the algorithm of brainwave frequency is inversely related to brainwave amplitude. A healthy display is when the amplitude of Theta is about 1.7 times Beta, and Alpha is about 1.4 times Beta. This algorithm can be disrupted for many reasons and understanding the disruptive dynamic is important. If Beta amplitude is greater than Alpha or Theta, it can result from Beta amplitude being too high or Theta or Alpha amplitudes being too low. In general, if the Theta/Beta ratio is over about 2.3 or so, probe for cognitive deficiencies and look for similar ratio at Cz. If the Theta/Beta ratio is low, below 1.2 or so, probe for stress tolerance issues and look for deficient Theta/Beta at O1. The latter can be because Theta amplitude is low or because Beta amplitude is too high, or both. Elevated Beta amplitude is associated with problems with stress tolerance, anxiety, sleep problems, and other sequellae of poor stress tolerance. Elevated Theta tends to be more cognitive slowness rather than cognitive functioning being affected by anxiety. Elevated Alpha amplitude, generally indicated by Theta/Alpha ratios below about 1.0, is indicative of the high-frontal-Alpha form of ADHD, a most pernicious form of the attention deficiencies. Probe for problems with planning, organizing, sequencing, and following through on tasks. Most critical, with this form of ADHD, also probe for problems with emotional dysregulation. If Alpha amplitude is blunted, that is below Beta; this can be associated with hypervigilance associated with exposure to severe emotional stressors. Blunted Alpha is most often found in cases where there are also trauma markers at Cz, O1, or both locations.

Once satisfied that the amplitude/frequency algorithm is satisfactory, the imbalances in the frontal regions are evaluated. Again, with three brainwave bands at two sites, the combinations that are possible are numerous. Beta, if elevated in the right relative to the left probe for dysphoric mood states; if elevated in the left probe for anxiety conditions; elevated bilateral Beta, as stated above, probe for hyper-vigilance, poor stress tolerance, anxiety, and anxiety-based depressed mood states.

Alpha, if elevated in the left relative to the right probe for dysphoric mood states and, in particular, probe for reactive depression; if elevated in right relative to the left probe for mood volatility, defiance, and interpersonal difficulties; if elevated bilaterally probe for cognitive deficiencies, attention problems, and emotional dysregulation.

Theta, if elevated in left relative to the right follow same probes as for Alpha left elevation; if elevated in right probe for mood volatility; if elevated bilaterally probe for attention difficulties, cognitive slowing (particularly with seniors).

It is important to keep in mind that shadow symptoms should be considered as well. Client with imbalances under the clinical threshold guidelines are important for understanding the subtleties of the client's emotional state. Combined brainwave amplitude configurations likewise are important to consider such as elevations of both Alpha and Theta, perhaps both below clinical threshold, that may be associated with fibromyalgia, viral infections, Lyme's, and the like.

At location Fz: Elevated Delta, probe for cognitive deficiencies. If trauma markers in evidence (locations Cz and/or O1), elevated Delta may be emotional blunting. Pain patients also often have Delta elevations.

Elevated HiBetaGamma (HBG) (28–40 Hz) and Beta (16–25 Hz) are associated with perseverative thought processes. When the ratio of HBG/B is high, above 0.60 or so, probe for stubbornness, preservative thought processes, and compulsive behavior patterns. Interestingly, this elevation can have positive features as well. In Optimal Performance programs, the ratio is often kept high (0.60 to 0.70) to facilitate willfulness, determination, and perseverance, but the client is always advised to be mindful of potential for inflexibility. When the sum of the amplitudes of HBG and Beta is high, above about 15, clients frequently report fretting, worry, and stuck cognitions which can be events that have occurred, tasks that have to be accomplished, or songs that keep playing in their head.

The ratio of LoAlpha (8–9 Hz) to HiAlpha (11–12 Hz) and Alpha Peak Frequency (APF) are indicators of brain efficiency. When the Lo/HiAlpha ratio is high, above about 1.50, probe for cognitive inefficiencies, emotional dysregulation, and vulnerability to physical disorders such as colds, flus, and the like. For clients with serious challenges, cancer for example, increasing brain efficiency is usually included in any neurotherapy program given data indicating relationship to immune functioning.

Once the clinician has made note of all of the clinical indicators outlined above, considering as well, any that might be shadow symptoms, suppositions are formed as to the cognitive and emotional state of the client. The suppositions include some hypotheses about the broader experiential climate to which the client may be or have been exposed. Children, for example, who show a trauma marker at Cz, a reactive depression marker, and an emotional volatility marker may well be prime candidates for bullying. Likewise, children who show poor stress tolerance markers, an ADHD marker, and a trauma marker may be unhappy, easily frightened, indifferent, frequently ill, have sleep problems, and poor self-esteem. This goes beyond the actual data but is a frequent qualitative picture of children struggling with poor academic performance, sleep problems, and joylessness.

As is evident from the correlations with the client's self-reported symptoms at intake, both between items on the checklist as well as between symptoms and EEG measures, there are many associations that can be helpful in developing a comprehensive and insightful understanding of the client's condition. The associations reported in this book were based on correlations of 0.30 or greater. This arbitrary threshold was selected so that the associations were not only statistically significant (with a sample size around 1,000, very small coefficients can be statistically significant) but clinically meaningful. Coefficients of 0.30 or greater mean that the shared variance is about 10 % or greater, so these associations can provide useful clinical information.

In addition to the associations, both among symptoms and between symptoms and ClinicalQ EEG measures, there are associations between the EEG measures that are interesting as well as potentially helpful to the clinician. The Theta/Beta ratios, for example, are correlated between the locations. Between Cz and O1 ($r=0.50$); Fz ($r=0.46$); F3 ($r=0.47$) but interestingly with F4 ($r=0.26$). F4 and O1 Theta/Beta also correlates low again at $r=0.26$. The correlations between F3 and F4 for Alpha ($r=0.91$), Beta ($r=0.87$), and Theta ($r=0.20$) indicate that the Theta bandwidth is associated with these low correlations of Theta/Beta among the sites with location F4. The differences between the correlation coefficients between F3 and O1 versus F4 and O1 are both statistically reliable ($z>3.0$, $p<0.002$) as are the differences between the correlation coefficients for F3/F4 Theta versus those for Alpha and Beta ($z>20.0$, $p<0.0001$).

It is interesting to recall that Theta amplitude at location F4 is more responsive to negative mood states, viral infections, medications, and conditions like fibromyalgia, chronic fatigue, and Lymes's disease as compared to the contralateral F3 location. In addition, there are no clinically significant correlations among any of the frontal imbalance measures. Thus, imbalances in Alpha, Theta, and Beta are independent of each other. However, as was discussed previously, client's self-reported symptoms do correlate in ways suggestive of misattribution of causality. For example, there are significant correlations between any of the depression markers and self-ratings of items indicative of negative mood states. There are also significant correlations between markers for anxiety and self-rated anxiety but also for depressed mood states. That is, clients may rate themselves as depressed and anxious but only show EEG markers for anxiety. The relationship is between the client's attitudes not the frontal EEG markers.

Another interesting factor grouping is the correlations between SMR amplitude at location Cz and the Theta/Beta ratios at other brain sites. The Theta/Beta correlations with SMR at Cz are all positive O1 (0.38), F3 (0.34), F4 (0.48), Fz (0.78), whereas the correlation with summated HighBetaGamma plus Beta amplitudes is negative (−0.40). All correlations are reliable ($p<0.001$). This would be consistent with SMR amplitude up-training to enhance quiescence in general and as an alternative to Beta amplitude down-training should the clinician find the latter not efficient.

There are several important reasons for starting any therapeutic relationship with the ClinicalQ. First, it permits the therapist to approach treatment in a no-nonsense, data-oriented fashion. Clients are shown data that are associated with their presenting complaints. This is done rapidly and candidly. It is not business as usual, in which they have to endure long drawn out intake procedures with a therapist who may or may not understand their situation. Compare this with a situation in which after 6.5 min of recording data the therapist is able, with remarkable accuracy, to tell the client the exact nature of the complaints for which that person has sought treatment. Equally as important, the therapist can show the client exactly what is going to be done to treat the complaints.

A client is anxious and depressed (which the therapist has told the client, not the other way around) and the therapist shows the client what the neurotherapy is going to correct. In this case, it might be that the Theta/Beta ratio at O1 was 0.85 and the right frontal (F4) Beta was 35.2 % greater than left frontal (F3) Beta. I would have said to this client that the deficiency in the back of the brain is "often associated with poor stress tolerance, general anxiety, can't shut your brain off, sleep quality problems, predisposition to self-medicating behavior, and a worn-out form of depression." The frontal disparity in Beta would be explained as a predisposition to depressed mood states. Overwhelmingly, the wide-eyed client responds affirmatively to these probes, occasionally denying one of the symptoms (e.g., sleep quality issues).

Second, as implied in the above, the ClinicalQ shows the therapist and the client where treatment is to be focused. No hit-or-miss, no protocols based solely on client report, and no general pot-boiler canned protocols that generally show some benefit to most everyone because of brain stimulation and copious doses of placebo.

Third, and in my judgement most important, the ClinicalQ allows the therapist to see elements of cognitive/behavioral deregulations that are not frank disorders. Worded in another manner, this procedure frees the therapist from the absurdity of DSM diagnostic procedures. A special section of the *Journal of Abnormal Psychology* (2005) examined many of the problems with the categorizing diagnostic system, and the authors suggested dimensional models as an alternative. If we look at the procedure for applying the label of ADHD, we see that for the label ADHD (inattentive type) one must demonstrate that the child manifests at least six out of a list of nine symptoms. For the label "predominately hyperactive/impulsive type," the child must be rated as manifesting at least six out of a list of nine symptoms plus three other conditions. What if the child shows only five, or for that matter, one of the symptoms? In short, this system, like some psychological testing, affords no useable data to guide therapeutic decisions. A child may find school difficult because he has a minor excess of Theta amplitude at location Cz, a mild Theta deficiency at location O1, and a mild Beta amplitude excess at location F4 relative to location F3. This child could be characterized as having minor manifestations of attention deficiency, racing thoughts, and depression, none of which would survive the diagnostic categorization. This child might be thought of as having shadow symptoms of several disorders that in combination are causing the difficulties in school. Treatment proceeds in a data driven orderly fashion of normalizing the minor deviations from normative ranges as determined by the ClinicalQ.

The fourth, and perhaps most important, benefit of the ClinicalQ is that it permits a form of therapy not dissimilar to Cognitive Behavior Therapy (CBT). The organizing concept of CBT is that it changes the client's view of the world. It changes how a person speaks to himself/herself and it changes his/her core emotional belief. Feedback from the ClinicalQ provides many of these same benefits. The person is shown the neurological bases for their complaints, and importantly they are empowered to take corrective action to change their life. Their depression, for example, is predisposed because of a neurological condition that is correctable.

Career dead ends may be the result of an untreated form of ADD that predisposes a person to have severe difficulties with focus, concentration, retention of information, planning, organizing, sequencing, following through on tasks, and with motivation. These neurological conditions are correctable, so behavioral change is facilitated. The person can discard their self-disparaging beliefs that they are losers, deficient, and worthless failures. They can also discard the fatalistic notion that they were simply given a bad deal in that they have genetic deficiencies that make them losers.

The elegance of the ClinicalQ system lies in the simplicity of the procedure. One is analyzing raw data not filtered through databases. Minor deviations from normative ranges are readily observable and the potential for negative synergy of these minor departures can be analyzed. The latter is often completely missed in other diagnostic systems because the modest departures do not survive statistical criteria for significant deviations. In short, far from being less precise than the full QEEG with database comparisons, the ClinicalQ often provides far more sensitive data alerting the therapist to the qualitative texture of the client's difficulties. It is for this very reason that I strongly disfavor computerized assessment software that interprets miniQ data. The purpose of the ClinicalQ is to avail oneself of data obscured by the full QEEG normative databases. The computerized analysis systems for miniQ data seem to be an effort to develop a poor therapist's QEEG. This is entirely the wrong use of the ClinicalQ. The ClinicalQ provides data obscured by the full QEEG databases, and in my clinic, we virtually always have a ClinicalQ even though many of our clients eventually have a full QEEG.

Clients with conditions such as simple ADD (Swingle 2001), depression, sleep problems, and many anxiety disorders are assessed with the ClinicalQ, proceed to treatment immediately, and rarely require a full QEEG. Because of the specificity of the ClinicalQ data and aggressive braindriving treatment protocols (Swingle 2003 Summer), discussed in later chapters, these clients complete treatment in well under industry averages. The rapidity of treatment is also largely the result of the profound confidence the client develops in the efficacy of neurotherapy because of their experience of the ClinicalQ intake procedure. And these interpretations are based on systematically collected reliable data that can make sense to any client.

Chapter 3
Treat the Condition Not the Label

As has been stated several times, neurotherapy blends perfectly with other treatment modalities and metaphors. Neurotherapy closes the gap in many therapies in that the clinician will be able to attend to the biological component of treatment. Neurotherapies, in any of the many manifestations and methodologies, including neurofeedback and neuroguided stimulation (braindriving), are NOT stand-alone treatments. They are simply not adequate, on their own, to treat any meaningful clinical condition. Further, if one is truly treating the condition and not the label, then any one-size-fits-all procedure is also simply inadequate.

One-size-fits-all neurotherapies do, however, come in many guises if not sizes. "Dynamical" models of treatment purport that if one gives the brain a good shake-up or workout, there will be a general reorganization tending toward normative, state-sturdy baselines. And like all notions about interconnected systems, there is some theoretical, if not empirical, merit to this position.

Serious scientist/practitioners working with database-guided therapies (e.g., z-score training) do show that interconnectivity among brain sites become more "normalized" with such treatments. We do know that improved connectivity is associated with client reports of improved functioning with traumatic brain-injured clients. So there may be some merit for including shake-the-pot sessions as part of neurotherapy packages for some clients. But, there is scant evidence for shake the pot as a one size fits all for all clinical clients. As stated previously, departures from normative functioning need not be associated with any clinical complaint. In fact, such departures from the "normal" may be associated with unique skills and approaches.

Most of the flagrantly bogus one-size-fits-all franchise-like enterprises feature some form of shake the pot. Some, however, are a bit more sophisticated and have specific shake-the-pot protocols for specific label complaints such as depression and ADHD. Symptom-based protocols are much too imprecise for reasons already stated. This lack of precision is apparent regardless of whether or not the base treatment metaphor is shake the pot or treating (activating or quieting) presumed brain regions associated with the condition or on general notions such as relaxation/quieting protocols benefit everyone.

P.G. Swingle, *Adding Neurotherapy to Your Practice*,
DOI 10.1007/978-3-319-15527-2_3

However, with clinical populations, there are specific comprehensive neurotherapy protocols that can have general beneficial effects for many clients. These protocols have emerged from clinical practice and clinical databases. The efficacy of these general protocols is based on QEEG data indicating neurological commonalities among clinical clients.

General Protocols

Stress Tolerance Increase the Theta/Beta ratio in the occipital region of the brain (sites O1 and O2). This protocol emerged from the early work of Gene Peniston (Peniston and Kulkosky 1999) who demonstrated that increasing the amplitude of Theta and Alpha at the back of the brain had substantial beneficial effects with chronic hospitalized alcoholics. The "Alpha/Theta" protocol has been found to have benefit with clients with other complaints as well.

The Theta/Beta ratio can be enhanced with several protocol variations. The original Alpha/Theta training protocol is to initially increase Alpha amplitude and then switch over to increasing Theta amplitude. Variations on this protocol include going directly to increasing Theta amplitude and/or decreasing Beta amplitude. The latter is particularly effective when the client's Theta/Beta ratio is low because of elevated Beta and less the result of deficient Theta amplitude.

The reason that increasing the Theta/Beta ratio has general beneficial effects for many clients is because over 70 % of clinical clients (in our sample population) have a Theta/Beta deficiency in the occipital region of the brain. Further, that percentage increases to over 80 % for clients diagnosed with bipolar disorder. The "emergency" braindriving protocol, described in Chap. 6, includes Theta enhancement.

Clinicians must be mindful that increasing the Theta/Beta ratio can have the effect of "releasing" blunted Alpha which is related to emotional trauma. In our database, about 40 % of general clinical clients show a trauma marker, and this percentage jumps to a stunning 87 % with clients diagnosed with a bipolar disorder. Hence, client receiving this "relaxation" therapy may have an abreactive episode when the emotional content associated with traumatic events surface during the treatment. This emotional abreaction has been described by many clinicians who train up Alpha and/or Theta amplitude posteriorly.

Clinicians working with other forms of relaxation therapies have also commented on relaxation-induced panic episodes with clients. Clinically, of course, these releases are very therapeutically beneficial, and clinicians frequently use such procedures for precisely this purpose. However, these potential effects of such training further emphasize that only licensed healthcare professionals should be practicing in these arenas. Further, there are going to be some potentially harmful outcomes from the unlicensed practitioners who include this generally beneficial protocol into their one-size-fits-all programs.

Body Quiescence Based on the seminal work of Barry Sterman (Sterman and Egner 2006; see also Robbins 2000) on the treatment of seizure disorders, protocols for increasing the sensory motor rhythm (13–15 Hz) amplitude over the sensory motor cortex (locations C3, Cz, and C4) have been shown to have a generally beneficial effect on decreasing physical arousal. Often this training includes simultaneous reduction in the amplitude of Theta as well. SMR training has been shown to improve sleep quality (Hoedlmoser et al. 2008), motor tics (Tansey 1986), hyperactivity (Lubar and Shouse 1977), and pseudoseizures (Swingle 1998).

Brain Brightening Cognitive functioning is generally improved when the amplitude of slow-frequency EEG is reduced (cf. Abstra-Angelakis et al. 2007; Swingle 2002) over the frontal cortex or the sensory motor cortex. This can be accomplished in several ways including reducing the amplitude of EEG activity in the 3–9 Hz range or by increasing the peak frequency of Alpha (8–12 Hz). There are several variations in these brain-brightening protocols such as reducing Theta amplitude while simultaneously increasing Beta (16–25 Hz) amplitude. Some protocols focus on just increasing Beta amplitude, others on reducing Theta. Bandwidth of the slow frequency varies as well with some clinicians preferring to focus on Theta and others on low Alpha (8–9 Hz), and some prefer to train across the entire bandwidth (3–9 Hz). Decreasing Delta (1–3 Hz) likewise can have a cognitively brightening effect.

Although there are occasions when clinicians may find it beneficial to use one of the generic protocols, listed above, in general one should always rely on QEEG-guided treatment. Clients who arrive in states of severe arousal and angst may be too distraught to proceed with obtaining a reliable QEEG, whether the ClinicalQ or more extensive full-head EEG. In such circumstances initially administering either the stress tolerance or the body quiescence protocol (infrequently both) may be the most efficacious way to commence therapy with the client. Braindriving protocols described in Chap. 6 are very effective for rapidly quieting such distressed clients.

Very frightened children and very confused elderly clients, likewise, are often best started with a generic protocol to both introduce them to treatment setup as well as to facilitate quieting. It should be noted that some straightforward peripheral biofeedback protocols to reduce muscle tension, improve breathing, increase blood flow, and the like may be equally efficacious for quieting the distraught client prior to commencing more thorough EEG assessments.

Infants are another example of clients that may be best treated initially with generics. For example, children with infantile seizure disorders such as West Syndrome may respond best with generic body quieting (Theta/SMR) protocols coupled with careful monitoring of seizure activity.

Anxiety

The Great Smoky Mountain Study that began in the early 1990s was a longitudinal study of childhood psychiatric disorders. The study provided significant data on the development and stability of these disorders over time. The research sample was large consisting of three cohort groups of about 1,400 children each. The children were 9, 11, and 13 years at baseline. They were assessed up to 11 times between the ages of 9 and 26. There were some unforeseen and interesting changes in the economic environment that indicated that as poverty went down, so did the incidence of psychiatric problems in young people.

There are many interesting findings associated with the study. For example, it was found that 13 % of subjects met the criteria for a psychiatric disorder in any 3-month period during the assessments. Based on these periodic measurements, the researchers estimated that the cumulative prevalence of a DSM-4 psychiatric disorder was 61 % by age 21 with an additional 21 % displaying subclinical psychiatric problems. This indicates that, by their estimates, about 82 % of young people had psychiatric problem by the age of 21. Focusing only on the anxiety disorders, it was estimated that by the time the subjects were in their mid-20s, about 25 % of the participants met the criteria for an anxiety disorder (Copeland et al. 2014).

Given the magnitude of the problem of anxiety disorders in children, finding efficacious treatment is obviously a top priority. It is in this arena that neurotherapy shows such efficacy. By using an evaluative system, such as the ClinicalQ, the putative mechanism associated with the disorder can be identified. At the basic clinical level, the conditions are assessed, speedily, by looking at regions of the brain and treating the inefficiencies in functioning. Unfortunately, much research in this area is what is called "horserace" designs. Whether double blinded and placebo contrasted or not, they are nonetheless designed to see which treatment wins the race. Many rely on patient subjective reports which, although important, do not determine if the putative mechanism has been altered.

This problem is nicely shown in the series of studies on the treatment anxiety disorders in children. As shown in Fig. 3.1, the efficacy of sertraline and Cognitive Behavior Therapy (CBT) is about equally effective with about 50 % positive response rate that is about twice as effective as the placebo. If combined, however, the improvement is about 80 % clearly indicating that, at 12-week follow-up, the combination is the preferred treatment (Cummings et al. 2013). After 6–9 months, however, we see that all treatments are equally and substantially effective with about 80 % positive response rate (Piacentini 2014). So, the general message from this horserace is that after 6 months or so, it does not really matter which treatment is used. Unfortunately, we do not have sufficient placebo data, so we cannot say anything about placebo effectiveness at 6 months.

At 6-year follow-up, however, the data indicate that all treatments have equivalent relapse rates, of about 50 %, and presumably young adults with chronic and lifelong disorders (Ginsburg et al. 2014). That our treatments are not very effective is further suggested by studies of hospitalization and, more importantly, rehospitalization rates. Hospitalization rates for adolescents with psychiatric diagnoses have increased by 42 % over a 10-year period as reported by Bladder (2011). Further, rehospitalization rates, in Arnold et al. (2003) analyses, were in the 30–50 % range.

The problem, in short, is that we have been treating labels not the neurological condition.

The strategy of treating the condition and not the label is shown in the case example in Fig. 3.2. This client, a 51-year-old female, has a long history of "depression" that has not responded efficiently to any treatment, psychological or pharmaceutical. The problem is this client does not have depression markers; she is

CBT, SERTRALINE, AND COMBINED THERAPY ALL SHOW DURABILITY FOR TREATMENT OF ANXIETY FOR YOUTH

TREATMENT	FOLLOW-UP	POSITIVE RESPONSE RATE %
CBT	12 weeks[a]	59.7
SERTRALINE		54.9
COMBINED		80.7
PLACEBO		28.3
CBT	24- 36 weeks[b]	80.0
SERTRALINE		82.0
COMBINED		83.0

AT A SIX YEAR FOLLOW UP THERE IS A 50% RELAPSE RATE IN THE LONG-TERM EFFECTIVENESS OF SERTRALINE AND CBT TREATMENT [c]

Fig. 3.1 Treatment of anxiety disorders in children. *Sources*: (**a**) Cummings et al. (2013), (**b**) Piacentini (2014), (**c**) Ginsburg et al. (2014)

CZ	VALUES
EO Alpha	8.12
EC Alpha	9.58
% Change EO to EC Alpha > 30%	18.02
EO Alpha Recovery	8.95
% Change EO - Alpha Recovery	10.29
Theta Amplitude EO	10.58
Beta Amplitude EO	12.00
EO Theta/Beta	0.88
Theta Amplitude Under Task (UT)	10.90
Beta Amplitude UT	19.39
UT Theta/Beta	0.56
% Change T/B EO to T/B UT	-56.38
% UT Beta Increase	60.93
Total Amplitude	33.42
Theta Amplitude preceding Omni	12.36
Theta Amplitude with Omni	11.97
% Change in Theta with Omni	-3.22
Alpha Peak Frequency EC	9.9
Alpha Peak Frequency EO	9.6
Theta/SMR EC	1.70

O1	VALUES
Alpha EO	5.82
Alpha EC	5.64
% Change in Alpha EO to EC	-3.11
EO Alpha Recovery	4.33
% Change EO - Alpha Recovery	-34.24
Theta Amplitude EO	4.98
Beta Amplitude EO	7.57
Theta/Beta EO	0.66
Theta Amplitude EC	4.20
Beta Amplitude EC	3.53
Theta/Beta EC	0.49
% Change T/B EO to T/B EC	-34.65
Alpha Peak Frequency EC	10.2
Alpha Peak Frequency EO	10.5

F3 & F4 (ALL EC)	VALUES		% Difference F3-F4
F3	F3	F4	
Beta Amplitude EC	21.5	22.0	2.5
Alpha Amplitude EC	8.0	9.2	15.1
Theta Amplitude EC	7.3	9.2	27.0
EC Theta/Alpha	0.34	0.42	23.9
EC Total Amplitude	36.8	40.5	10.0

FZ (ALL EC)	VALUES
Delta (2 Hz)	4.5
HiBeta Amplitude	21.6
Beta Amplitude	19.2
HiBeta/Beta	1.12
LoAlpha/HiAlpha	0.91
Alpha Peak Frequency	9.9

Fig. 3.2 Client with anxiety-based depression

"depressed" because her life is in shambles resulting from severe anxiety and poor stress tolerance, identified in less than 15 min by a basic ClinicalQ assessment.

Following the ClinicalQ probes, the client has trauma markers at both locations (Cz and O1), marked bilateral elevation of frontal Beta, marked deficiency in the Theta/Beta ratio at O1, poor sleep quality marker also at O1, marked elevation of 16 Hz through 40 Hz at Fz, emotional volatility marker at F4, and very good brain efficacy marker at Fz. All of these neurological conditions are a perfect storm for severe anxiety conditions. She is "depressed" because she cannot cope.

A female client in a hospital-based day program had a very similar ClinicalQ profile to the one shown in Fig. 3.2 above. She had major trauma markers at both locations, marked deficiency in the Theta/Beta ratio in the occipital region, marked elevation of frontal Alpha amplitude, as well as elevated 16–40 Hz amplitude at Fz.

This young woman was diagnosed with "pseudoseizure disorder," often also called non-epileptic seizure disorder. Pseudoseizures are presumed to be sequelae of exposure to severe emotional trauma and may be related to the flashback process (see Swingle 1998a, b). In short, the pseudoseizure, which can be fainting, fugue-like state, tremors, and full-blown myoclonic like seizures, may occur to block the severe emotional distress associated with emotional flashback. The trigger for the emotion-blocking seizure may be physiological arousal as appears probable from the data shown in the following Fig. 3.3.

During treatment sessions, seizures were common occurrences. This client had significant multiple medications, many to be used Prn, which was a major complicating factor in her treatment. During neurological/physiological and/or psychological/behavioral treatment sessions, this client's physiological signs were

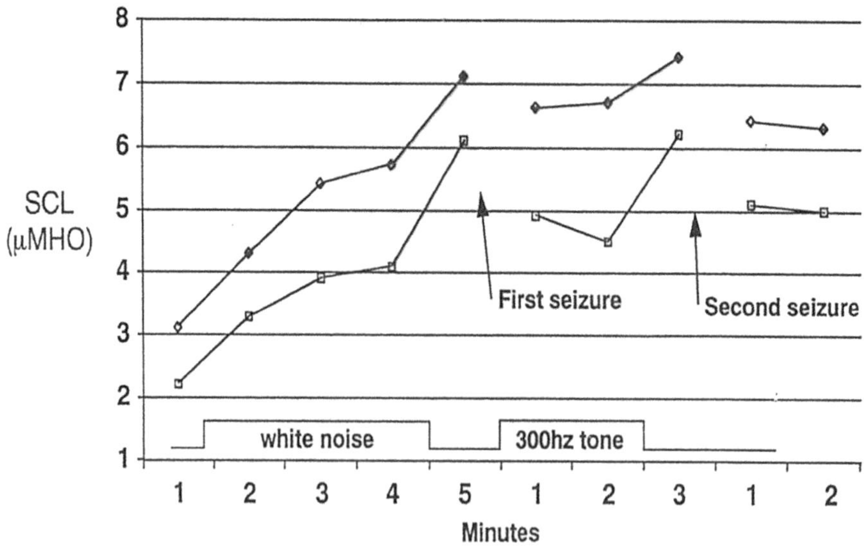

Fig. 3.3 Electrodermal conductance during auditory stimulation of a client with pseudoseizure disorder

monitored including electrodermal conductance, electromyographic amplitude (frontalis placement), peripheral blood flow (finger placements), heart rate, and blood oxygen saturation.

As shown in Fig. 3.3, seizure activity occurred when the electrodermal conductance rose above 6 micromhos bilaterally. The figure shows provoked activity associated with contingent sound (client's tolerance of feedback and conditioned stimuli sounds to be used in neurotherapy was being evaluated), but similar physiological patterns were found in therapy sessions when strong emotion was elicited. Many readers will be familiar with the use of electrodermal (GSR) monitors during psychotherapy sessions to identify emergence of emotional content that may be important.

Depression

A common complaint of clients we all treat is "I'm depressed." The client has a huge array of options for receiving treatment for this amorphous condition including prescription medications, supplements, exercise, endless psychotherapies, R & R, and of course an array of neurotherapies. In the latter case, we have normative database guided; neurofeedback, the z-score zapping paradigms (brain site-specific frequency amplitude departures penetrating z threshold evoke an infinitesimal amp/gauss zap), and z-score neurofeedback; sLORETA; canned feedback protocols based on defined condition (i.e., "depression"); and franchises with proprietary symptom checklist-driven canned protocol systems.

ClinicalQ-based treatment is different. The cases, described below, exemplify how treatment is guided by bottom-up assessment and verification. Neurotherapeutic protocols are then precisely targeted at these verified neurological inefficiencies. The ClinicalQs for the following cases are presented in summary form rather than the full output, as shown above. In addition, only data relevant to the present discussion are included in the summary.

The fundamental neurological condition one finds in depression is an imbalance in the frontal cortex with the right (F4) being more active as compared with the left (F3). The data presented in the previous chapter indicate that negative emotional states including feelings of depression, worthlessness, negative emotional life, nothing to look forward to in life, and fearfulness are all related to EEG data indicating that the right frontal cortex is more active than the left. There is substantial evidence for this relationship. An excellent review of the literature supporting the relationship between depression and elevated activity of the right relative to the left hemisphere (Hecht 2010) also reviews the evidence for comorbid conditions related to this imbalance as summarized in the abstract:

> Depression is associated with an inter-hemispheric imbalance; a hyperactive right-hemisphere (RH) and a relatively hypoactive left-hemisphere (LH)... There is evidence that the RH is selectively involved in processing negative emotions, pessimistic thoughts and unconstructive thinking styles—all which comprise the cognitive phenomenology of

> depression and in turn contribute to the elevated anxiety, stress and pain associated with the illness. Additionally, the RH mediates vigilance and arousal which may explain the sleep disturbances often reported in depression. The RH had also been linked with self-reflection, accounting for the tendency of depressed individuals to withdraw from their external environments and focus attention inward. Physiologically, RH activation is associated with hypercortisolemia, which contributes to the deterioration of the immune system functioning and puts depressed patients at a greater risk of developing other illnesses, accounting for depression's high comorbidity with other diseases. Conversely, the LH is specifically involved in processing pleasurable experiences, and its relative attenuation is in line with the symptoms of anhedonia that characterize depression. The LH is also relatively more involved in decision-making processes, accounting for the indecisiveness that is often accompanied with depression (Hecht 2010).

The imbalance between the right and the left frontal regions can result from several neurological conditions as measured with the EEG. The Davidson (1992) pattern, identified years ago, is when Alpha has greater amplitude in the left relative to the right. However, there are many other conditions that result in this imbalance. For example, the client shown in Fig. 3.4 is what we might call "garden variety" depression. This client has an imbalance where Beta is greater in the right relative to the left. Clinically this appears to be the "genetic" predisposition for depression although it is found in client's having recently experienced a loss. Figure 3.5 shows the Davidson depression marker of elevated Alpha in the left relative to the right frontal cortex. The client shown in Fig. 3.6 is similar in that Theta is greater in the left relative to the right resulting in the right being more active than the left. Clinically the two patterns just described (low-frequency amplitude greater in the left) are very frequently associated with reactive depression (exogenous). Finally in Fig. 3.7, we see a pattern often found with a person with the predisposition to depression who has experienced a severe emotional stressor that has triggered the predisposition.

Emotional trauma, exposure to a severe emotional stressor or an accumulation of emotional stressors, is associated with a blunting of the Alpha response at locations Cz and O1. We understand that this marker is associated with incompletely processed emotional sequelae of the emotional event(s). Exposure to emotionally negative images (corpses) has been shown to temporarily blunt the Alpha response and fortuitous exposure to severe emotional stress with clinical clients likewise revealed Alpha blunting. Alpha blunting is seen as restricted elevation of Alpha amplitude when clients close their eyes (Swingle 2013) (see the parameters for this response in the Appendix to this chapter). The Alpha response is completely ignored in the normative databases.

Occasionally one sees clients who report that they are depressed but there are no depression markers in the ClinicalQ. There are many profiles that are found but two are relatively common. The profile shown in Fig. 3.8 shows no depression markers but both trauma markers. There are other details of clinical relevance in this profile, but the critical point for this discussion is that unprocessed trauma can be manifested as reports of "depression." The lack of the reactive depression markers (e.g., Davidson 1992) may indicate that the client is in the numb phase of posttraumatic exposure. However, although of interest to speculate on these matters, clinically one

Fig. 3.4 "Genetic" depression

Cz	M Θ/β	α↑%	
	1.69	85.2	
O1	Θ/β O	Θ/β C	α↑%
	1.62	1.74	110.9
	Θ	α	β
F4	12.1	9.9	8.6
F3	11.3	9.2	7.1
%d	7.1	7.6	21.1
Fz	Dz	Hβ/β	Σ
	10.9	0.82	10.0

Fig. 3.5 Reactive depression (Alpha)

Cz	M Θ/β	α↑%	
	1.37	38.3	
O1	Θ/β O	Θ/β C	α↑%
	2.20	2.24	55.8
	Θ	α	β
F4	9.7	7.6	6.9
F3	9.2	9.3	6.3
%d	5.4	-22.4	9.5
Fz	Dz	Hβ/β	Σ
	8.9	0.52	11.2

Fig. 3.6 Reactive depression (Theta)

Cz	M Θ/β	α↑%	
	1.48	59.3	
O1	Θ/β O	Θ/β C	α↑%
	2.02	1.74	75.4
	Θ	α	β
F4	9.7	9.1	6.3
F3	14.0	8.2	6.1
%d	-44.3	10.9	3.3
Fz	Dz	Hβ/β	Σ
	8.8	0.61	12.6

proceeds to release the Alpha and then utilize whatever therapy the clinician judges relevant to resolve the condition. It is with these trauma clients that the one-size-fits-all franchisers are the most destructive. Often one will hear comments about how to quiet an emotionally abreacted client who has been subjected to one of the canned protocols, exactly the opposite of good clinical practice.

Fig. 3.7 Trauma-triggered depression

Cz	M Θ/β	α↑%	
	2.24	10.9	
O1	**Θ/β O**	**Θ/β C**	**α↑%**
	1.53	1.47	55.8
	Θ	**α**	**β**
F4	11.8	7.7	8.9
F3	11.7	6.7	6.6
%d	1.0	14.9	34.8
Fz	**Dz**	**Hβ/β**	**Σ**
	7.5	0.58	7.5

Fig. 3.8 Trauma-based depression

Cz	M Θ/β	α↑%	
	1.49	8.1	
O1	**Θ/β O**	**Θ/β C**	**α↑%**
	1.55	1.64	15.4
	Θ	**α**	**β**
F4	13.0	8.5	6.6
F3	14.4	8.9	6.7
%d	-10.8	-4.7	-1.5
Fz	**Dz**	**Hβ/β**	**Σ**
	11.7	0.74	13.6

Fig. 3.9 Anxiety-based depression

Cz	M Θ/β	α↑%	
	1.34	39.6	
O1	**Θ/β O**	**Θ/β C**	**α↑%**
	1. 06	0.87	64.8
	Θ	**α**	**β**
F4	12.8	9.7	6.9
F3	12.0	8.9	10.6
%d	6.7	9.0	-53.6
Fz	**Dz**	**Hβ/β**	**Σ**
	7.3	0.77	11.4

The profile shown in Fig. 3.9 is also quite common. These are clients in severe states of anxiety who feel hopeless, frightened, and out of control. They report being "depressed" because their lives are in shambles, or they feel they are going to decompensate, or they feel just plain helpless. Treating these conditions with anti-depressants is a formula for creating a lifelong problem. The ClinicalQ identifies the areas for neurotherapeutic treatment quite precisely. Again, there are several other

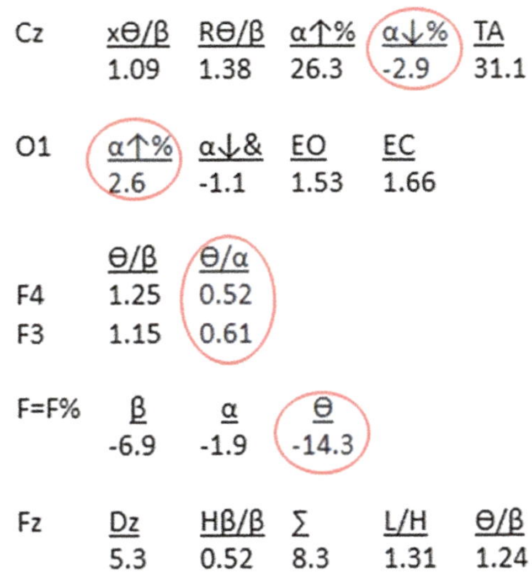

Fig. 3.10 High frontal alpha-based depression

aspects to this EEG profile of clinical relevance such as markers for cognitive perseveration, but for the purposes of the present discussion, it is the two markers of deficient Theta/Beta ratio at the occipital location and elevated left frontal Beta that identify the anxiety state.

As noted in earlier sections, clients who rate themselves high on "depression" have, on average, 10 % lower amplitude Theta/Beta ratio at location O1 relative to those clients who rate themselves not depressed ($t=2.20$, $p<0.03$, $df=367$). In addition, the correlation between the ratings of "I feel depressed" and "I am very anxious" is 0.51 ($p<0.0001$, $df=912$), indicating that many clients who report depression may well be experiencing the sequelae of severe anxiety without any of the neurological markers for depression. In our experience at the Swingle Clinic, these are the clients who frequently report histories of many years of "depression," many years of therapy, and many different pharmaceutical cocktails. Obviously, neither the therapies nor the pharmaceuticals were satisfactory; otherwise they would not be seeking treatment. The problem, again, is that the treatment of these clients was unsuccessful because the label not the neurological condition was being treated.

Another common profile associated with client complaint of "depression" is associated with misdiagnosed and mistreated high frontal Alpha form of ADHD (see Fig. 3.10). This case will be reviewed more thoroughly in the next section. The depression associated with this condition is reactive because the client feels out of control, emotionally dysregulated, and disheartened. Frequently and unsuccessfully treated with a variety of psychotherapies and/or pharmaceutical cocktails usually including both antidepressants and anxiolytics (and often with atypical antipsychotics as well), these clients often have treatment histories that span decades. As the above ClinicalQ profile indicates, this client's major neurological condition is marked excessive Alpha amplitude over the frontal cortex. It is ADHD, in other words, and this client would have been spared decades of angst if the correct condition, not the label, had been treated.

The treatment of children with early signs of depression can be particularly challenging. In the first instance, it is very likely that the indicators will be missed or interpreted as some other condition such as anxiety, ADHD, and even mild autism. Depression in children is often not associated with outward indicators of sadness that we associate with depression. These children often seem to be lacking energy, interest, and motivation. They do not appear interested in the activities in which they are engaged. However, these characteristics can also be related to sleep problems or anxiety. As detailed in the last chapter, children with deficient Theta/Beta ratios in the occipital region of the brain are more likely to be rated, by a parent, as having a sleep problem and lower in self-esteem. They are also rated higher on "unhappy," "poor self-esteem," "indifferent," "frequently ill," and "easily frightened."

Many of the above characteristics can also be considered symptoms of depression. In a study of preschoolers (Luby et al. 2014), children diagnosed with depression were 2.5 times more likely to be diagnosed with major depression disorder at school age. However, the authors note that preschool depression does not meet the criteria for major depression disorder. They suggest that onset of preschool depression may be more common than is clinically recognized. These children show lack of joyfulness during normal play rather than frank sadness, and the symptoms appear to be intermittent. This is related to the finding from the ClinicalQ database indicating that children with the low Theta/Beta ratio at the occipital site show more "indifference" which seems consistent with the lack of joyfulness reported by Luby et al. (2014).

The above data make it quite clear that one should treat the putative neurological condition and not the symptoms or diagnostic label. Anxious and sleep-disturbed children may show many of the signs of depression, as do adults, and be inappropriately treated for depression. Following the neurological data from the ClinicalQ directs treatment to the functional brain inefficiency, regardless of label, that can be treated to improve the client's condition.

In addition to the relationship between reported anxiety and reported depression, anxious clients also rate themselves higher on fatigue ($r=0.39$), perseverative thoughts ($r=0.47$), negative view of their future ($r=0.40$), irritability ($r=0.39$), problems with concentration ($r=0.33$), and feelings of worthlessness ($r=0.45$). These associations are quite consistent with the correlations with self-rated depression: fatigue ($r=0.52$), perseverative thoughts ($r=0.42$), negative view of the future ($r=0.56$), irritability ($r=0.38$), and problems with concentration ($r=0.37$). In addition, self-rated depressed clients are more likely to rate themselves as feeling physically unwell ($r=0.36$). All of the correlation coefficients are statistically significant ($p<0.0001$, $N=914$).

Recall the data on manifestation of neurological predispositions such as in the study of monozygotic twins, one of whom had manifested schizophrenia, whereas about 50 % of the twin did not. Depression markers are indicators of predisposition. They are markers for neurological conditions that can manifest to clinical level depression. But many will not. This is one of the principal reasons why normative databases are notably inaccurate at detection of clinical conditions, whereas clinical databases are considerably more useful for the clinician. However, even in clinical populations, some clients presenting conditions other than depression might also have markers for unmanifested conditions. Clients with no markers for depression distribute themselves about equally among low, mid, and high self-ratings on the depression items on the intake questionnaire. About 32 % rate themselves as high, 34 % as mid-range, and 33 % as low on "I feel depressed." Alternatively, 26.3 % of clients with at least one depression marker rate themselves as without depressed mood states. These are the clients with neurological markers that, like the unmanifested genetically predisposed schizophrenic, have not been exposed to conditions that result in symptom manifestation.

Bipolar Disorders

Many clients come with diagnosis of "bipolar" disorder. When questioned, many state that they have a history of depression but no recall of any "manic" phases. Others feel that the hyper states have been the primary cause of their difficulties in all aspects of their life. In keeping with the therapeutic dictum of "treat the condition not the label," the ClinicalQ is used to identify neurological conditions that may predispose a client to depressed, agitated, and emotionally dysregulated states. Clients may report symptoms of depression resulting from feeling hopeless, powerless, or stupid because of irrational behavior and emotional states associated with the manic phases in some forms of bipolar disorder. On the other hand, bipolar diagnoses have been attached to conditions that are actually high frontal Alpha forms of ADHD.

From the clinical database, 23 clients came for treatment with a diagnosis of "bipolar disorder" from an independent psychiatrist. Of this group of clients: 91.3 % had one or both of the trauma markers (blunting of the Alpha response at locations Cz and O1) as compared to 39.9 % in the general clinical group ($z=6.77$, $p<0.001$, $N=891$); 87.0 % had at least one of the three emotional volatility or dysregulation markers (elevated Alpha amplitude at F3 and F4, elevated right frontal Theta amplitude at F4, or elevated right frontal Alpha amplitude) as compared to 68.3 % in the general clinical group ($z=2.03$, $p<0.05$, $N=891$); 82.6 % had the poor stress tolerance marker (deficient Theta/Beta ratio at O1) as compared to 71.4 % in the general clinical group ($z=1.18$, *ns*); 58.0 % had at least one of the four depression markers (elevated F4 Beta amplitude, elevated F3 Theta and/or Alpha amplitude, elevated Theta/Beta ratio at F3) as compared to 37.0 % in the general clinical group ($z=2.01$, $p<0.05$, $N=891$). It is interesting to note that these data are not inconsistent with common pharmaceutical treatments for these conditions that often include mood stabilizers, antidepressants, and anxiolytics. It is also interesting to note that the principal discriminators for the bipolar group were the trauma markers and the markers for emotional volatility and dysregulation. About 90 % of the bipolar clients had trauma markers, and about the same percentage had an emotional dysregulation marker. Further 100 % of this group had at least one of these markers.

About half of the bipolar clients had at least one marker for depression as compared with about a third of the general clinical group. It is apparent then that the major discriminative neurological features of the bipolar group are emotional volatility markers and indicators of exposure, past and/or present, to severe emotional stress.

There also appears to be an elevated connectivity among brain sites. Correlations between frontal sites F3 and F4 for Theta, Alpha, and Beta amplitude, the ratios of Theta/Beta and Theta/Alpha, and correlations between these frontal sites and the SMR at location Cz were all substantially higher in the bipolar group as compared with the general database. Of the 17 correlations, 16 were greater (direction ignored) for the bipolar group (binomial probability, $p<0.001$). The difference between the average correlations for the general group ($r=0.29$, SD=0.16) and for the bipolar group ($r=0.79$, SD=0.21) is statistically significant ($t=6.26$, $p<0.001$, $df=20$). The coefficients are also significantly different (recognizing that these are averages, direction ignored) based on sample size of 16 ($z=3.66$, $p<0.001$).

There was a nonsignificant trend for a greater proportion of the bipolar group to have markers for poor stress tolerance which was high for both groups. In this regard, it is interesting to note that adolescents diagnosed with a bipolar disorder have a higher probability of developing a substance use disorder (SUD), most frequently cannabis. In a sample of bipolar adolescents hospitalized with mania, 48 % had or developed an SUD (Stephens et al. 2014). This high rate of SUD is consistent with the high rate of deficient Theta/Beta ratios found in our sample of clients diagnosed with a bipolar disorder.

It is also apparent that the neurology is not the only area of concern in dealing with these clients. As is discussed throughout this book, the efficient processing of the sequelae of exposure to severe emotional stress (trauma) is central to the effective treatment of these clients. Similarly, some focus on developing self-regulation procedures for dealing with emotional dysregulation is central. This is particularly problematic because these dysregulated behaviors are likely to developed stability because of conditioning. The common example is the emotionally volatile individual who's unpredictable and explosive emotional tirades have been reinforced by being instrumental to the control of others.

Two clients, both of whom were diagnosed as bipolar, showing different ClinicalQ patterns are shown in the following two figures. Figure 3.11 shows the trauma marker at Cz, the deficient Theta/Beta ratios at O1 (with the sleep quality problem marker), the frontal depression marker (elevated right frontal Beta), and two emotional/mood volatility markers (elevated right frontal Theta and Alpha amplitudes).

The second case, shown in Fig. 3.12, is the rare bipolar client that does not show trauma markers. This client rated herself at maximum scale levels for depression, anxiety, fatigue, perseverative thoughts, feelings of worthlessness, and problems with concentration and sleep. This client has the high frontal (F3 and F4) Alpha amplitude that is associated with both cognitive and emotional dysregulation.

These individuals have problems with planning, organizing, and following through and problems with concentration and focus. They also often have major

CZ	VALUES
EO Alpha	5.11
EC Alpha	5.07
% Change EO to EC Alpha	-0.71
EO Alpha Recovery %	-4.74
EO Theta/Beta	1.85
UT Theta/Beta	1.67
% Change T/B EO to T/B UT	-10.66
Total Amplitude	17.04
Alpha Peak Frequency EC	9.5
Alpha Peak Frequency EO	8.7
Theta/SMR EC	2.32

O1	VALUES
Alpha EO	3.79
Alpha EC	10.49
% Change in Alpha EO to EC	176.78
EO Alpha Recovery %	17.66
Theta/Beta EO	1.35
Theta/Beta EC	1.02
% Change T/B EO to T/B EC	-32.35
Alpha Peak Frequency EO	10.7

F3 & F4 (ALL EC)	VALUES F3	VALUES F4	% Difference F3-F4
Beta Amplitude	3.67	4.41	20.08
Alpha Amplitude	4.61	6.05	31.40
Theta Amplitude	5.98	7.63	27. 54
Theta/Beta	1.83	1.74	5.2

FZ (ALL EC)	VALUES
Delta (2 Hz)	6.30
HiBeta/Beta	0.63
Sum HiBeta + Beta	8.08
LoAlpha/HiAlpha	0.74
Alpha Peak Frequency	10.0

Fig. 3.11 Female, 37 years old, client diagnosed with bipolar disorder

CZ	VALUES
EO Alpha	11.3
EC Alpha	16.4
% Change EO to EC Alpha	45.1
EO Alpha Recovery %	8.0
EO Theta/Beta	1.78
UT Theta/Beta	2.79
% Change T/B EO to T/B UT	56.4
Theta/SMR EC	1.35

O1	VALUES
Alpha EO	10.0
Alpha EC	28.3
% Change in Alpha EO to EC	183.0
EO Alpha Recovery %	28.0
Theta/Beta EO	1.73
Theta/Beta EC	1.09
% Change T/B EO to T/B EC	37.0

F3 & F4 (ALL EC)	VALUES F3	VALUES F4	% Difference F3-F4
Beta Amplitude	7.1	8.5	19.7
Alpha Amplitude	13.6	12.1	12.4
Theta Amplitude	8.7	11.5	32.2

FZ (ALL EC)	VALUES
Delta (2 Hz)	6.0
HiBeta/Beta	0.42
Sum HiBeta + Beta	11.2
LoAlpha/HiAlpha	1.59

Fig. 3.12 ClinicalQ summary of 51-year-old male diagnosed with bipolar disorder

problems with emotional dysregulation with irritability, mood swings, and volatility. The profile also shows marker for sleep disturbance (deficient eyes closed Theta/Beta ratio at O1), depression (elevated Beta amplitude at location F4), and an additional marker for mood volatility (elevated Theta amplitude at F4). This client also shows the marker for another form of ADHD and a particularly troublesome one. Note that the Theta/Beta ratio is in an acceptable range under at-rest conditions but jumps substantially when the client was under cognitive challenge (reading out loud). This is very problematic, for the brain, although seemingly within normal limits, produces substantial Theta amplitude when the client is attempting to focus. This is often associated with subjective feelings that conditions get worse the harder the person tries to concentrate (very discouraging for a school-age child).

Obviously the treatment for these two clients will be quite different. The first client is likely to have emotional abreactions when the Alpha response is restored as the emotional properties of the memories of the traumatic event start to emerge. Both clients have markers for depression and sleep problems, but the second client also has two markers for different forms of ADHD, one of which, as stated above, is also related to emotional dysregulation. One often sees clients with major depression complaints who show these ADHD markers but often no depression markers. This is usually associated with problems with life discouragements including academic, career, and interpersonal relationships. The "depression" is associated with the feelings of failure, despair, helplessness, hopelessness, and confusion. These clients often do not respond well to antidepressant medications and often have long histories of psychotherapy and psychopharmacology. The lack of meaningful progress with these therapies further contributes to feelings of despair and confusion.

The Attention Deficit Hyperactivity Disorders

In this section, we cover the disorders that are, indeed, disorders of attention. In this category we examine the neurological conditions that directly affect attention and hyperactivity. These are situations in which the symptoms are not primarily the result of some other condition such as depression. Much has been written about various forms of ADHD, and we find that researchers and clinicians differ in the number they suggest. Most of these variations in forms of ADHD are really ADHD plus various comorbid conditions such as sleep disturbance, depression, oppositional behavior, anxiety, and the like. As the reader will find, the labels and "types" of ADHD are largely irrelevant. From the perspective of "bottom-up," we look at the neurology of the child and correct relevant anomalies in functioning.

In latter chapters, the conditions that interfere with a child's ability to be attentive in school but are not neurological disorders of attention are reviewed. These will include conditions of poor stress tolerance, predisposition to depression, oppositional and defiance disorders, and frightened and traumatized children.

One of the problems we have with the statistics associated with consequences of untreated ADHD is that the methods for diagnosing these conditions are so flawed. As pointed out in an earlier chapter, the top-down method for diagnosis of attention deficiencies is simply inappropriate. However, with this in mind, let us remember some of the sequelae of untreated attention problems.

There is disagreement among researchers about the risk factors associated with untreated ADHD. Part of this problem, of course, is the fact that ADHD is a "wastebasket diagnosis." However, most of the disagreement is not about the fact that untreated ADHD leads to life complications; rather, that this disagreement centers on the extent of the risk. And as we shall review at various times throughout this book, different forms of ADHD pose different risks for individuals who remain untreated into adulthood. Other factors, of course, are important, including any psychological comorbidity one might have such as depression and anxiety, as well as gender and culture, to name but a few.

Table 3.1 Sample studies of adult populations with untreated ADHD conditions

ADHD-associated risks
Social/emotional/addiction problems
Alcoholism and/or drug addiction 50 %
Mood or anxiety disorder 60 %
Twice as likely to be divorced
Criminal behavior
Twice as likely to have been arrested
Prison inmates 45 % ADHD [general population (GP) 1.9 %]
Police contact: children 5.7 times greater; adults 10.8 times greater than GP

Although there are some inconsistencies in the data, nonetheless a relationship between untreated ADHD and criminality seems clear. Data collected on incarcerated males indicate much higher proportions of those with ADHD-like behaviors than in the general population. Interestingly, these individuals are not only more likely to be charged with a crime and arrested, but they are also more likely to be indicted and far more likely to be imprisoned. Perhaps this simply indicates again that they lack the capability for responsible planning, organizing, sequencing, and monitoring their personal situation once they have been charged with a crime.

A study, by Dr. Ginsberg and colleagues, of long-term male inmates in a Swedish prison found that 40 % had ADHD and less than 7 % had ever been diagnosed with this condition. Another study, by Drs. Fletcher and Wolfe of Yale University, of 13,000 adolescents over a long time period found that those with ADHD were twice as likely to commit a robbery and 50 % more likely to have sold drugs, as compared to their peers.

So, it seems clear that undiagnosed and untreated ADHD is a very substantial risk factor for criminal, and otherwise irresponsible, behavior. The challenge is to make sure that we treat the behaviors that are causing the trouble and not be corralled by the label we put on a specified grouping of these troublesome behaviors. Doing the latter markedly reduces our success rate for helping children overcome these hurdles to successful and fulfilling lives.

The data shown in Table 3.1 come from various studies of adults with untreated ADHD (Biederman et al. 2006; Kessler et al. 2006; Rösler et al. 2004; Young et al. 2002). And although one can quibble about the magnitude of some of these findings, nonetheless the data are striking. The following table gives some statistics from various studies of the consequences of untreated ADHD. This is a table of adult populations of individuals whose ADHD was either not diagnosed properly and/or did not receive proper and efficient treatment for the condition.

Comorbid mood and anxiety disorders are very common with ADHD. The lifetime comorbidity has been estimated at 80 % in individuals with ADHD (Goodman 2007). This is not surprising considering the effects of untreated ADHD on adults. Many of these individuals have difficulty staying in school and/or training programs, sustaining relationships, and sustaining employment. They have problems with planning, organizing, sequencing, and following through on tasks. Many of the clients we see, who live with ADHD that was untreated, are in states of what we might call reactive depression or despair. Life is just not going well for them. Often they have been in multiple relationships and things are not going well in their present relationship. This is often directly related to their inability to plan ahead and organize their lives. In addition, they usually have difficulty handling finances properly and trouble with participating in an organized and emotionally functional and rational relationship.

Hence these people frequently come for treatment complaining of depression when, in fact, it is reactive depression; they are depressed because of their life circumstances, not because of any neurological predisposition to depressed mood states, although, of course, they may have neurologically based depression as well.

These people are often extremely anxious as well. They may be in serious financial difficulty because of the ADHD affecting their careers and affecting their ability to manage finances properly. So, as shown in the above table, 60 % comorbidity of mood and anxiety disorders with ADHD is not surprising. We certainly see very high levels of comorbidity at the Swingle Clinic. So, we see both sides of this dimension: people who come in with a diagnosis of depression who are depressed because of the effects of ADHD and, alternatively, people who come in with a diagnosis of ADHD who are depressed with symptoms of lack of interest, poor motivation, and fatigue. The significant diagnostic precision of the ClinicalQ, as described by Susan Olding in a previous chapter, allows us to accurately isolate the areas of the brain causing the problems. We can then, in turn, develop neurotherapy treatment protocols that efficiently treat these conditions. The label for the pathology is obviously of trivial importance.

The Chattering Brain

The data associated with risk of alcoholism and other addictions is not as clear-cut. Certainly, depression and anxiety, as mentioned above, might well lead to self-medicating behavior in which the person drinks to get some peace and forget his or her troubles. However, it could be a neurological condition associated with genetic predisposition to hyperarousal which is strongly related to vulnerability to alcoholism. This neurological predisposition turns up routinely in children and adults diagnosed with ADHD. Neurologically, this condition is indicated by a marked deficiency in the ratio of the strength of slow frequency (Theta) divided by the strength of fast-frequency (Beta) brain wave activity in the back of the brain. People with this condition in the back of the brain report that they have difficulty quieting themselves. They simply cannot find a switch to turn the brain off. People with this neurological pattern complain of poor stress tolerance, predisposition to anxiety, self-medicating behavior, sleep quality problems, chatter in the head, and fatigue. The deficient Theta/Beta ratio can be associated with either a deficiency in Theta amplitude or an excess of Beta amplitude, and sometimes both. As discussed in Chap. 1, the precision of the ClinicalQ initial EEG assessment provides precise data on the brain wave activity. Thus, we know if we need to increase Theta amplitude, decrease Beta amplitude, or both, to effectively and efficiently treat this condition.

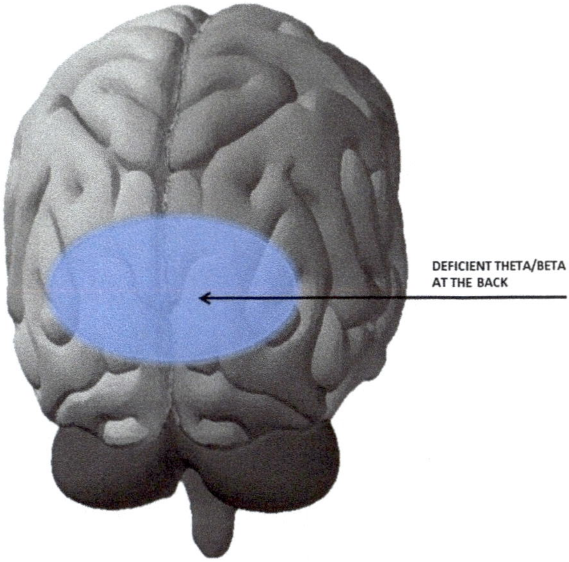

Fig. 3.13 Deficient Theta/Beta

It is interesting to note that the symptoms associated with the deficient Theta/Beta ratio in the occipital region are often quite different depending on whether the deficiency is related to excessive Beta or deficient Theta amplitude. The brain location implicated in this condition is shown in Fig. 3.13.

Children with this condition are routinely diagnosed with ADHD. And, as we have just discussed, in reality, this is a form of genetic predisposition to addictive behavior found in children diagnosed with an attention problem prior to any exposure to alcohol or other substances. In adult populations with this form of attention problem, we find the expected elevated levels of alcoholism and other substance addictions, including nicotine.

The child with this condition simply cannot sit still, experiences disconcerting brain chatter, has poor tolerance to stress, often has poor sleep quality, is very easily distracted, and often does not do well in school. Although diagnosed with ADHD because of poor focus, easy distractibility, and elevated activity levels, medicating this child with a stimulant will exacerbate the problem. Hence, although we prefer to treat this condition with neurotherapy without medications, nonetheless we consult with physicians for clients who prefer medication. In this condition, stimulants are contraindicated and alternative medications would be recommended.

The Hypoactive Brain (Inattentive)

Recognizing that there are many reasons why children cannot pay attention in school, many of which we will review in later chapters, we will start with a review of those neurological conditions that directly affect the child's ability to pay attention in school. Related to these conditions are conditions that are also associated

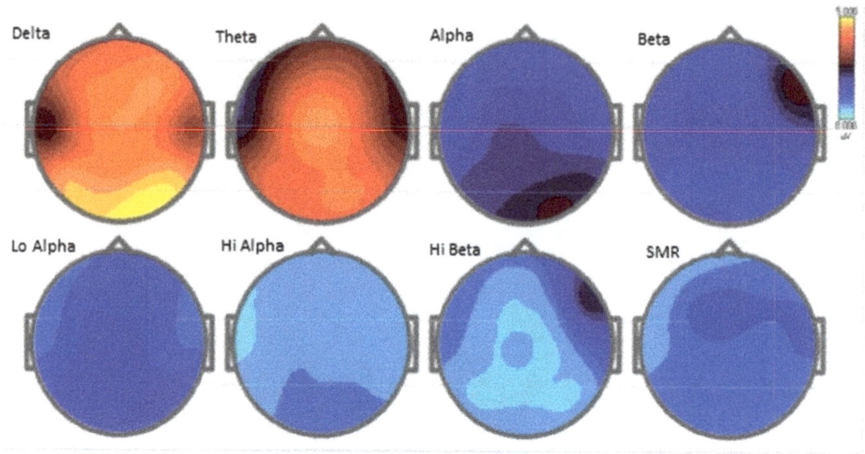

Fig. 3.14 Topograph of child with elevated Theta amplitude

with hyperactivity. In many circumstances, the brain wave pattern associated with an attention problem is also the one associated with the hyperactivity issue.

We start with what I call Common Attention Deficit Disorder (CADD). This is the least complicated form of an attention deficit disorder and the most easily corrected. It is also the form that responds most effectively to methylphenidate (Suffin and Emory 1995; Kuczenski and Segal 1997), but lasting improvement requires neurotherapy (Monastra et al. 2002).

As shown in Fig. 3.14, CADD is associated with elevated slow-frequency amplitude. Frequencies in the Theta range (3–7 Hz) are elevated, typically over the center and frontal regions of the brain but, as shown in Fig. 3.14, often over the entire cortex. When slow frequency is elevated in the brain, it means that those areas are hypoactive. These are the children who daydream a lot, simply cannot stay focused, are disorganized, and have very great difficulty staying on target.

In the best of all possible worlds, we see these children at a very young age. As I say in my workshops, a client directly from heaven is a little girl, perhaps 8 years of age, who has this simple form of CADD. Most importantly, she knows from the depth of her heart that the love of her parents for her is completely independent of any achievements she may attain. I can bet the farm that this child will respond very successfully to treatment and that treatment will likely only require between 15 and 20 sessions.

Just such a child is shown in Fig. 3.15. The initial data recorded at the intake assessment is shown on the top and labeled baseline. As you will note, the Theta/Beta ratio (the ratio of the amplitude of 3–7 cycles per second divided by the amplitude of 16–25 cycles per second) is 3.5. Anything above about 2.3 or so, with a child of her age, is usually indicative of an inattention issue. We would consider that this condition is of moderate severity.

The treatment for this is very straightforward. As described in the "Neurotherapeutic Treatment" chapter, the child is engaged in a video game that she

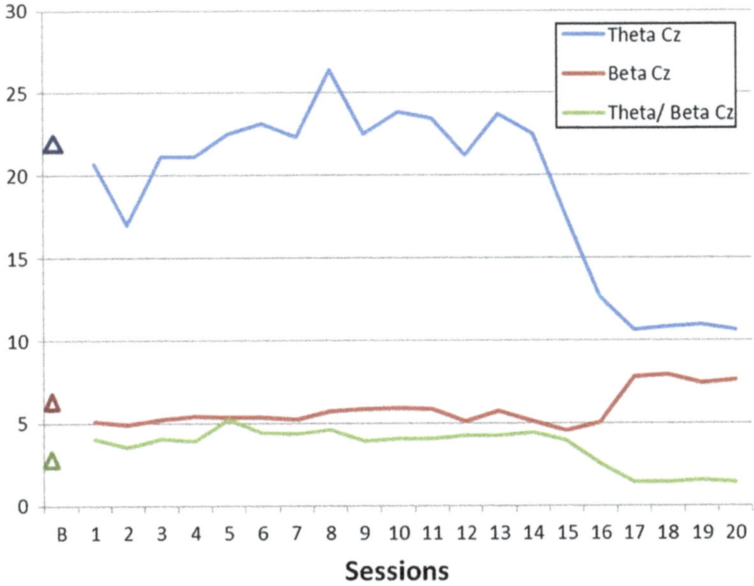

Fig. 3.15 Intake Baseline (B) and treatment progress of child with CADD. Baseline measures: *Theta* = 21.9 μV, *Beta* = 6.3 μV, *Theta/Beta ratio* = 3.5

plays with her brain. When the brain is doing what we want it to do, icons move on the computer screen, and this can be any one of a number of different games that are used for neuronal feedback.

Note that in the initial sessions the Theta/Beta ratio appears to be getting worse. She started at 3.5, but during the first 15 or so sessions, the ratio appears to be getting larger. This is not unusual that during the initial sessions the ratio appears to be getting worse. This may be related to the form of ADHD we reviewed in the initial chapter of the boy whose ratio became worse under challenge. Recall that the initial value shown on the baseline is an average value. When this child makes considerable effort during the treatment, then the ADHD condition worsens in many cases. It is very important for parents and the neurotherapist to understand that very often you get an increase in the symptom prior to symptom improvement. In this case, when we are challenging the child, the condition gets worse until after 18 sessions when she finally gets it. The Theta/Beta ratio drops markedly and is sustained for the final few sessions.

Figure 3.16 is a letter sent by the parents of this child. The important matter to note here is that the mother points out that the child, after a week of school, brought in a flute and played a solo in front of her classmates.

It is also interesting to note that this child changed schools so this was a completely new environment for her, and none of the classmates were familiar to her. But as the mother points out, she was not the least bit nervous, whereas in the previous year, before her treatment, it would have been impossible for her to perform in front of her classmates.

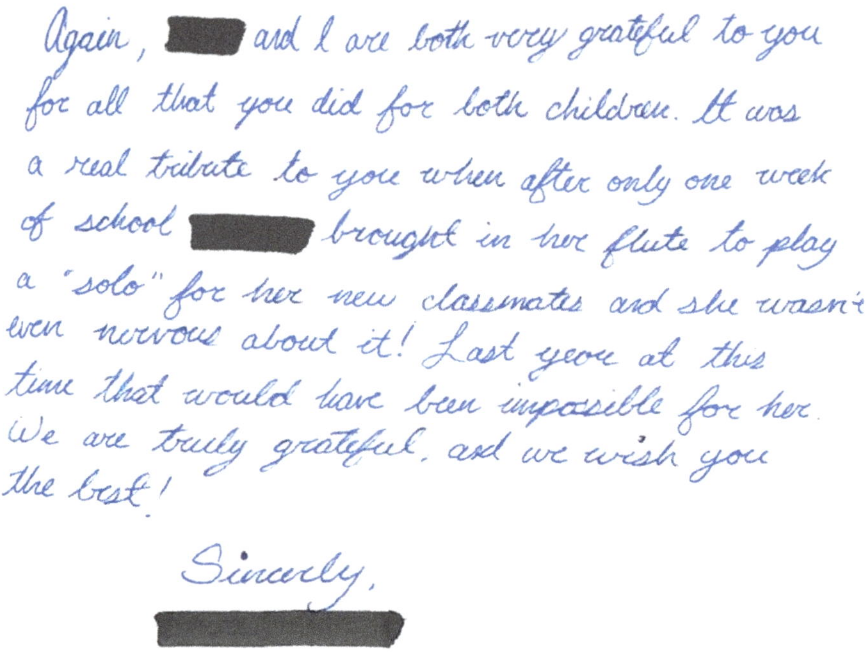

Again, ███ and I are both very grateful to you for all that you did for both children. It was a real tribute to you when after only one week of school ███ brought in her flute to play a "solo" for her new classmates and she wasn't even nervous about it! Last year at this time that would have been impossible for her. We are truly grateful, and we wish you the best!

Sincerely,

███

Fig. 3.16 Mother's letter regarding effects of neurotherapy for her daughter

What is important about this is that when you successfully treat ADHD, you also are treating the child's self-esteem. Children who have attention problems are very concerned about their performance. They see their classmates progressing in school with apparently much less difficulty than they are having. They question their intelligence, and they question their self-worth. Regrettably, if parents are not supportive, understanding, and helpful, but are instead judgmental, then the child's self-esteem suffers an even more severe blow. Once the ADHD was corrected, self-esteem was improved and she was able to perform her solo performance. As the saying goes "fix the child's self-esteem and you fix everything."

The Hypoactive Brain (Hyperactivity)

The difference between the inattentive and the hyperactive forms of ADHD is associated with two neurological factors. The first factor is a matter of degree. Common ADD, the form described above, is associated with elevated amplitude of slow-frequency brain wave activity primarily measured over the central part of the brain, but in general, it spreads out over most of the cortex. This is shown in the topographical maps of Fig. 3.14 in which Theta amplitude is seen to be elevated over the entire brain. At lower levels of elevated slow frequency, one gets inattentive

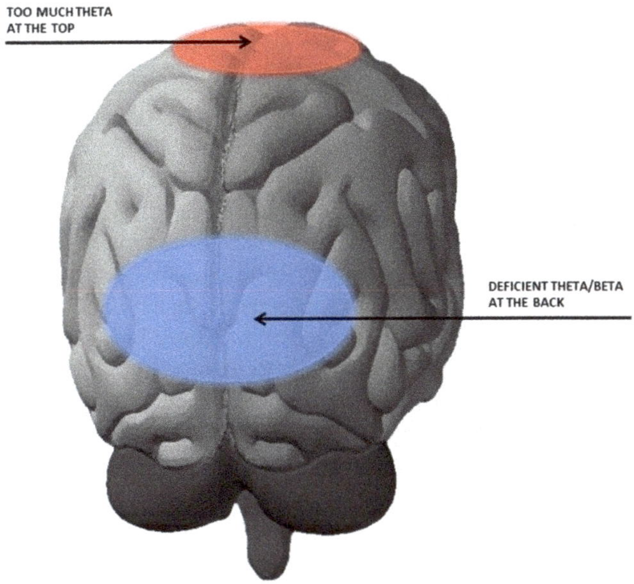

Fig. 3.17 Brain regions associated with hyperactive forms of ADHD

forms of ADD. These are the children that simply cannot stay focused and are easily distracted and prone to daydreaming, just like our little 8-year-old girl described earlier. At higher levels of excessive slow-frequency amplitude, the brain is seriously hypoactive and the child desperately needs stimulation. The hyperactivity is best conceptualized as self-medicating behavior. It is hard for us to appreciate the fact that sitting still is painful for the child. The movement activates brain activity principally over the sensory motor cortex, thus relieving the feelings of discomfort for the child. The primary areas associated with this elevated slow frequency are the central regions over the sensory motor cortex (the areas in the Fig. 3.17 outlined in red).

Occasionally, we have a complicating factor, such as a deficiency of slow frequency in the back of the brain. Deficiency of slow-frequency amplitude in the back of the brain is associated with poor stress tolerance, anxiety, and difficulty sitting still.

If we are only dealing with the issue of elevated slow frequency over the sensory motor cortex (the area directly on top of the head in Fig. 2.4), then stimulant drugs such as methylphenidate can be helpful because the drug stimulates the brain; hence, the child's need to self-medicate with hyperactivity is minimized. If, however, we have the complicating factor of a deficiency of slow-frequency amplitude or elevated fast-frequency amplitude in the back of the brain (i.e., low Theta/Beta ratio), then often drugs that are central nervous system stimulants, like methylphenidate, can exacerbate the problem.

The neurotherapeutic treatment of this condition is identical to the treatment of the less severe inattentive form. Basically, we decrease slow-frequency amplitude and/or increase the faster frequencies over the sensory motor cortex. The difference in treatment procedures for the "inattentive" ADHD child as opposed to the "hyperactive" ADHD child can be more than just a matter of degree. Again, depending on the age at which the child commences treatment, the ADHD child with the strong hyperactive component can be more of a behavioral problem in school and is likely being reinforced for highly disruptive behavior. This sets up a pattern of reinforcing disruptive behavior with disciplinary actions, such as sending the child to the principal's office, having the child go out in the hallway, or forcing the child to sit in an isolated corner of the classroom. A very sensible alternative to this procedure is the "safe room" which will be discussed in a subsequent chapter. For the present discussion, we want to keep in mind that the principal difference between the hyperactive and the purely inattentive ADHD child is more than simply a matter of degree. Because of the hyperactivity component, the child is likely to develop secondary problems, such as those just mentioned, because the child is being rewarded for disruptive behavior.

High Frontal Alpha ADHD

Too much Alpha in the front part of the brain can be a serious problem. We find this condition with many clients coming to the Swingle Clinic with diagnoses such as bipolar disorder, major depression, or the personality disorders. Cognitively, clients with high frontal Alpha forms of ADHD complain of problems with planning, organizing, sequencing, and following through on things. At the emotional level, individuals with high frontal Alpha also complain of problems with emotional flightiness, hyper-verbosity, and problems with emotional volatility, grounding, and consistency. This form of ADHD often responds most efficiently to serotonin-enhancing medications including SSRIs, SNRIs, and SARIs (Cipriani et al. 2009; Gunkelman 2014). Suffin and Emory (1995) report an 87 % response rate to antidepressants for clients with the high frontal Alpha form of ADHD.

It is also interesting to note that this is one of the conditions in which, historically, there has been discrimination against females in that male children received therapeutic attention more readily and systematically than females. The reason for this is that the female child with this condition was likely to be viewed as highly social, chatty, and flighty, but not too bright. The high frontal Alpha ADHD went undiagnosed because these behaviors and mood states were consistent with cultural negative stereotypes of female behavior. If diagnosed and treated properly at a young age, the lives of these children are literally saved.

Many adult females with this high frontal Alpha condition come to our clinic with their lives in shambles. Their relationships have not progressed adequately. They report having problems at all levels of their schooling, often dropping out prior to program completion. They have been unable to achieve their career aspirations. They feel emotionally unstable. The reason for their distress is pretty straightforward: these are the consequences associated with the high frontal Alpha form of

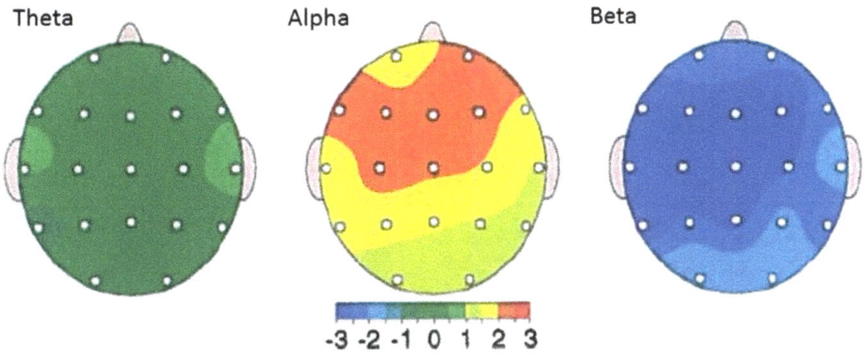

Fig. 3.18 Topograph showing distribution of Alpha brain wave amplitude of a client with high frontal Alpha ADHD

ADHD concomitant with the emotional and cognitive dysregulation characteristics of this condition. The brain area associated with the high frontal Alpha form of ADHD is shown in Fig. 3.18. As the topograph shows, the elevated Alpha is most pronounced in the frontal brain regions. Figure 3.18 shows the topograph output from an EEG of an actual client with a severe high frontal Alpha ADHD condition. Alpha, for this client, is elevated over the entire cortex but most prominently over the frontal cortex. Theta, shown on the left of the topograph is in normal range, showing in green. Beta, shown on the right of the topograph is somewhat deficient.

Alpha is like a parking frequency in the brain. Too much Alpha in the area of the brain associated with cognitive and emotional regulation results in these areas being hypoactive and, hence, cognitive and emotional dysregulation occurs.

High frontal Alpha becomes even more problematic when the person has other neurological predispositions for problematic conditions. These predispositions can include depression, poor stress tolerance, and perseverative thought processes. It is not difficult to understand how the Alpha dysregulation of emotional and cognitive functioning, when combined with predisposition to depression, poor stress tolerance, or anxiety, would be associated with diagnoses such as bipolar disorder or agitated depression.

Even without these other compounding conditions, individuals can be seen as emotionally unstable because of the emotional dysregulation factor. Frontal Alpha emotional dysregulation often results in individuals going in and out of depressed and/or agitated mood states. Combined with the cognitive dysregulation, these individuals have difficulty sustaining focus and problems with planning, organizing, sequencing, and following through on tasks. These combinations of emotional and cognitive difficulties give rise to substantial difficulties in school, work, social, and intimate relationship situations.

It is easy to imagine how the emotional dysregulation, often associated with chattiness, further gives rise to difficulties these children experience in school. They have trouble staying seated. They are always bouncing around, socializing with other children, and causing significant disruption in the classroom. These are the

a

Cz	xθ/β	Rθ/β	α↑%	α↓%	TA
	2.08	2.00	43.6	12.3	26.9

O1	α↑%	α↓%	EO	EC
	112.6	22.6	1.67	1.52

	β	α	θ	θ/β	θ/α
F4	7.9	14.4	6.2	1.27	0.54
F3	7.2	13.7	5.9	1.24	0.52

F=F%	β	α	θ
	5.1	5.1	9.7

Fz	Dz	Hβ/β	Σ	L/H
	5.7	0.58	12.5	0.67

b

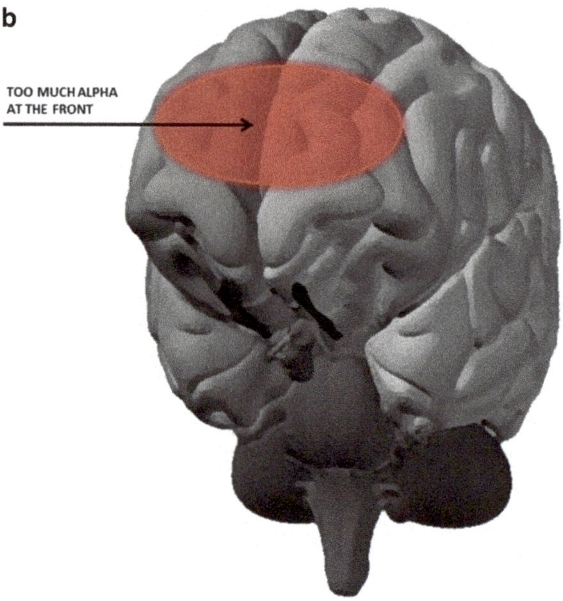

Fig. 3.19 (**a**) Data summary of electroencephalograph of a client with high frontal Alpha form of ADHD. (**b**) Brain areas associated with high frontal Alpha form of ADHD

children who will be talking to other children when they are supposed to be attending to the teacher. They have very great difficulty sustaining attention. One such case is shown in the following figures.

Figure 3.19a, b is an actual summary of the intake clinical EEG (ClinicalQ) of a young woman with high frontal Alpha form ADHD. The brain locations associated with these data are shown in Fig. 2.4. The data indicate that there are no significant inefficiencies in brain functioning other than a marked elevation of Alpha amplitude at locations F3 and F4, the frontal cortex. This is shown on the lines of data associated with F4 and F3. The ratio of Theta to Alpha is 0.54 at location F4 and 0.52 at location F3. The ratios should be closer to 1.50, or so, in each location; that is, the amount of Theta (amplitude of brain waves between 3 and 7 Hz) should be about 50 % greater than the amplitude of Alpha (8–12 Hz). This can also be seen in the amplitudes shown in lines F4 and F3. The Alpha amplitude is 14.4, almost twice the amplitude of Theta (7.9), and similarly, at F3, the Alpha is 13.7 and the Theta is only 7.2; (these amplitudes are in microvolts). The elevated frontal Alpha of this client is similar to that shown in topographical representation of the client shown in Fig. 3.18.

When this young woman presented for treatment, let's call her Jane, she seemed depressed and agitated. She teared up when she was describing how she felt her life was in chaos. She had just left a relationship that had been ongoing for 3 or 4 years and was in a job she considered boring and well below her level of capability. She just felt rotten. She had gone to see her physician on a number of occasions trying to describe her condition. Her physician felt that she was depressed and had prescribed antidepressants. In a condition such as this, antidepressants are obviously ineffective, short of sedation levels.

Jane, like many clients, was profoundly relieved to see that there was, in fact, a neurological reason for her chaotic, unfulfilled, and unfulfilling life. She went on to describe her early life in school in which her most profound memory was one of struggling to keep up. Everyone thought she was very sweet and nice but she clearly remembered feeling as though she was stupid. She simply could not keep up with the other children. Her parents were very supportive and patient and provided her with tutors to help her get through her homework. She just was not able to stay focused and was not able to plan and organize her daily activities. A poignant memory she related was of her going to her music lesson, having forgotten to bring her musical instrument, and feeling absolutely humiliated.

There were many such experiences that Jane related during the initial visit. She concluded by stating that her early childhood was simply miserable, and it was miserable not because her family was not supportive and loving but simply because she could not function properly in the school environment. The tragedy here is that a lot of this could have been prevented if she had been properly diagnosed at a young age. A simple 10-min brain assessment would have identified the problem, and a few very straightforward treatment procedures would have just simply changed her life.

It is a truism, of course, that the older we get, the longer it takes for the body and the mind to heal or to change. It is no different with neurotherapy. Treatment of an 8-year-old with Jane's condition would likely be resolvable in 15–25 sessions, whereas with Jane, more sessions are likely to be required. However, in addition to the possibility of a less plastic brain, there are other issues associated with dealing with older patients. The longer the condition has continued, the more failed relationships, the more failed jobs, and the more broken and shattered dreams. So in addition to the neurology, we have all of the psychological baggage that is associated with this form of ADHD: failure after failure after failure. If a client can really embrace the metaphor "look out the windshield, not the rearview mirror," then, of course, far fewer sessions are required to deal with the psychological aspect of this ADHD situation.

Jane was very fortunate she had a very high IQ. This is indicated by the very low ratio of slow to fast Alpha on the summary sheet (0.67). In addition, her brain functioning was quite within normal limits in all other areas with the exception of the high frontal Alpha. In short, we did not have a lot of other things that had to be corrected.

Jane finished in 22 sessions. She registered for a few courses to gain experience and regain her confidence at being able to do academic work. She got started on changing her life. This process took the better part of 3 years in which she got herself trained to pursue her dream of becoming a nurse. We saw Jane for follow-up visits four times during that 3-year period just to make sure that all of the neurological gains she had made remained stable. She felt that additional psychotherapy was not required, a sentiment with which I was in complete agreement.

Jane was lucky. She had a loving and caring family. She was very bright. The carnage associated with her high Alpha form of ADHD was not so overwhelming that she was not able to dig herself out and get on with her life once the neurological condition had been corrected. Although I do not have two cents worth of evidence to support this, my suspicion is that the reason she made out so well is because of the firm, loving, and structured family environment she had during the early years when she was suffering in school. Her core emotional belief about herself was not irrevocably destroyed by a sense of worthlessness. Jane was also very lucky in that other than the high frontal Alpha ADHD, she had no other significant brain wave inefficiencies. Many people are not as lucky as Jane.

Problematic Sleep Architecture

There are features found in the ClinicalQ that can help to identify not only that the person has a sleep problem, as discussed in the previous chapter, but also what features of the sleep architecture may be problematic. Client's self-ratings of "tired and fatigued" correlate with their ratings of having sleep problems ($r=0.36$, $N=914$, $p<0.0001$). However, client ratings of fatigue also correlate with self-rated depression ($r=0.52$, $p<0.001$) and self-rated anxiety ($r=0.39$, $p<0.0001$). In the latter cases, the problem may not be poor sleep or deficient sleep architecture. In fact, the problem may not be too little sleep but rather too much sleep which can result in feelings of continuous fatigue and tiredness.

In addition, ratings of being tired and fatigued also correlate with self-rated irritability ($r=0.30$), poor concentration ($r=0.38$), feeling unwell ($r=0.49$), and a group of ratings associated with depressed mood states including feeling depressed ($r=0.52$), low ratings of positive emotional life ($r=-0.36$), "nothing to look forward to" ($r=0.34$), and having negative and annoying thoughts ($r=0.29$). All of the correlation coefficients are statistically reliable ($p<0.001$, $N=914$, in all cases).

Clients at the Swingle Clinic who admit to a sleep problem often undergo a four-night sleep monitoring. These clients take an EEG-based monitor into their home environments and monitor their sleep over a four-night period. The Wireless Sleep (WS) assessment system (no longer commercially available) data correlate well with the ratings of Polysomnograph Raters (PR) scoring. Agreement between WS and PR scorings are in the range of 70 % (Pittman et al. 2004; Shambroom et al. 2011). The average correlations between the WS scorings and the PR scorings are equal to the correlations between the two PR scorings (between PR1 and 2, $r^{avg}=0.76$, SD=0.22; between WE and PR1, $r^{avg}=0.75$, SD=0.20; between WE and PR2, $r^{avg}=0.74$, SD=0.14). The meta-analyses indicate that there is higher agreement between the correlations of WE with either PR1 (WP1) or PR2 (WP2) with the PR1/PR2 (P12) correlation than the average P12 correlation itself (WP1/P12, $r=0.82$; WP2/P12, $r=0.81$; P12, $r=0.76$). The differences among the correlation coefficients are not significant ($z=0.3$, $p>0.5$).

Typically clients who show the deficient Theta/Beta ratio are first treated with neurotherapy to improve the deficiency in the occipital region in the brain. If they do not report improved sleep after a few sessions, a sleep assessment is often prescribed.

The following two figures show the results of just such a sleep assessment. In Fig. 3.20 the sleep assessment of a person with deficient REM sleep is shown, and in Fig. 3.21 an individual with deficient DEEP sleep is shown. In both of these cases, the client has inadequate total amount of sleep with a number of awakenings and long periods of wakefulness.

Data from clients treated specifically for deficient REM indicate that a poor Alpha response at location O1 is often associated with this deficiency. Data were obtained from clients who had four-night sleep monitoring. Those with total REM sleep of less than 60 min were compared with clients with adequate REM but with other sleep disturbances. Those with inadequate REM had an average Alpha

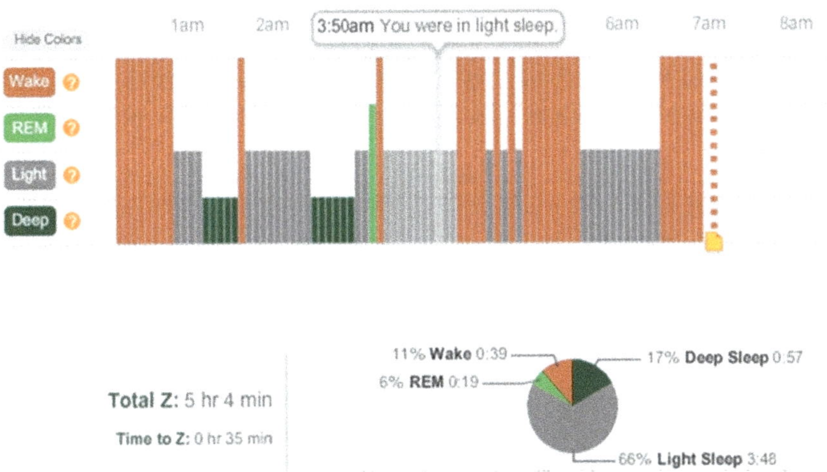

Fig. 3.20 Sleep record of client with adequate deep sleep but deficient REM and excessive waking

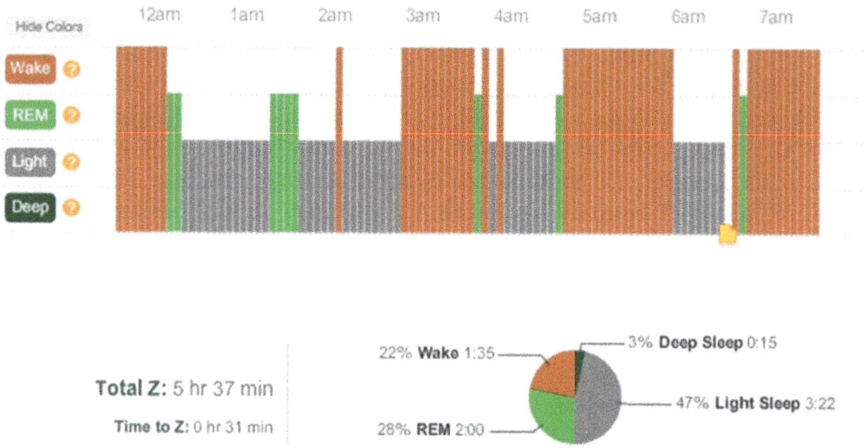

Fig. 3.21 Sleep record of client with adequate REM but deficient deep sleep and excessive waking

response of 28.1 %; those with good REM architecture had an average Alpha response of 121.9 % ($t=3.65$, $p<0.01$, $N=11$).

Poor deep sleep appears to be directly related to deficient Theta/Beta ratio at O1. The correlation between the Theta/Beta ratio and total deep sleep time was 0.32 ($p<0.02$, $N=59$) for the eyes open measurements and 0.43 ($p<0.001$, $N=59$) for the eyes closed condition. This is consistent with more frequent reports of sleep problems; when the eyes closed, Theta/Beta ratio is lower relative to eyes open measures. Interestingly, neither of the Theta/Beta ratios correlates with Total Sleep Time or REM Sleep Time ($r<0.1$ in all cases). Poor deep sleep also is related to the increase in Alpha amplitude when clients close their eyes. Clients with good deep sleep (between 50 and 70 min per night) had an average increase in Alpha amplitude of 83.3 % ($t=2.10$, $p<0.05$, $df=20$) as compared with those with poor deep sleep (less than 20 min per night) who had an average increase of 53.9 % ($t=0.92$, *ns*).

Divided on the basis of the Theta/Beta ratio, sleep-monitored clients with eyes open Theta/Beta ratios over 1.6 had an average deep sleep time of 86.5 min, whereas those with ratios below 1.00 had an average deep sleep time of 48.1 min ($t=2.78$, $p<0.01$, $df=25$). For the eyes closed condition, clients with Theta/Beta ratios over 1.60 had a mean deep sleep time of 101.7 min as compared with those clients with Theta/Beta ratios below 1.00 where the average deep sleep was 44.6 min ($t=4.06$, $p<0.001$, $df=35$).

A low Theta/Beta ratio can result from low amplitude of Theta or high amplitude of Beta or a combination of both amplitudes. It appears that for deep sleep the major determinant is Theta amplitude. The correlation between deep sleep time and Theta amplitude is 0.44 ($p>0.001$, $N=59$), whereas the correlation with Beta amplitude is 0.03 (*ns*).

The Identification and Treatment of Emotional Trauma

Bullying is a serious problem, and in one recent case, the child was terrified but equally frightened to tell a parent or teacher because of the bully's threat to hurt the child if he revealed the problem. Figure 3.22a shows the brain wave assessment of this child who was suspected to be a victim of bullying. In Fig. 3.22a, the area highlighted in red, showing the blunting of Alpha at a location directly in the center of the head, is a marker often associated with individuals who have been exposed to severe emotional stressors. Whenever we see this in a very young child, the two things that come to mind are bullying and family conflict. The second remarkable feature in this child's EEG, also shown in Fig. 3.22a, is a mild elevation of the Theta/Beta ratio over the center part of the brain. These ratios are in the range of 2.40, and anything above 2.2, or so, is associated with attention problems. In this case, we have a child in which we have a minor marker for an attention problem, but more importantly, we have a marker that indicates that this child has been exposed to emotional stress.

Moving on to Fig. 3.22b, we see that there is a very large disparity in the Alpha amplitude in the frontal cortex with Alpha being considerably stronger in the left relative to the right. As discussed in a previous chapter, this is a marker for depressed

a

CZ	VALUES	% CHANGE
EO Alpha	8.61	
EC Alpha	10.23	
% Change EO to EC Alpha > 30%		18.78%
EO Alpha Recovery	9.27	
% Change EO - Alpha Recovery		7.63%
Theta Amplitude EO	15.76	
Beta Amplitude EO	6.50	
EO Theta/Beta	2.47	
Theta Amplitude Under Task (UT)	13.69	
Beta Amplitude UT	5.89	
UT Theta/Beta	2.32	
% Change T/B EO to T/B UT		-6.45%
% UT Beta Increase		-10.29%
Total Amplitude	30.65	
Theta Aplitude preceding Omni	14.42	
Theta Amplitude with Omni	13.15	
% Change in Theta with Omni		-9.68%
Alpha Peak Frequency EC	10.00	
Alpha Peak Frequency EO	9.80	
Theta/SMR EC	3.15	

O1	VALUES	% CHANGE
Alpha EO	6.16	
Alpha EC	12.06	
% Change in Alpha EO to EC		95.84%
EO Alpha Recovery	5.70	
% Change EO - Alpha Recovery		-8.16%
Theta Amplitude EO	10.09	
Beta Amplitude EO	5.17	
Theta/Beta EO	1.95	
Theta Amplitude EC	10.46	
Beta Amplitude EC	6.99	
Theta/Beta EC	1.50	
% Change T/B EO to T/B EC		-30.21%
Alpha Peak Frequency EC	10.00	
Alpha Peak Frequency EO	9.90	

b

F3 & F4 (ALL EC)	VALUES		% Difference F3-F4
	F3	F4	
Theta Amplitude EC	10.10	16.93	
Beta Amplitude EC	6.37	7.06	
EC Theta/Beta	1.59	2.41	
% Diff F3T/B - F4TB EC			50.93%
Theta Amplitude EC	10.10	16.93	
Alpha Amplitude EC	13.47	9.28	
EC Theta/Alpha	0.75	1.83	
EC Total Amplitude	29.95	33.26	
*F4><F3 Beta	6.37	7.06	10.74%
*F4><F3 Alpha	13.47	9.28	-45.20%
*F4><F3 Theta	10.10	16.93	67.56%

FZ (ALL EC)	VALUES
Delta (2Hz)	10.05
HiBeta Amplitude	3.89
Beta Amplitude	6.15
HiBeta/Beta	0.63
Sum HiBeta + Beta	10.04
LoAlpha Amplitude	5.20
HiAlpha Amplitude	3.61
LoAlpha/HiAlpha	1.44
Alpha Peak Frequency	9.40

Fig. 3.22 Brain wave assessment of a bullied child

mood states. When the disparity is in the Alpha brain wave range, we have found that this depressed mood state is likely to be experiential in nature (i.e., reactive) as opposed to neurological.

Another brain wave feature shown in the ClinicalQ is a major imbalance in the amplitude of Theta in the front of the brain, where the right is considerably greater than the left. Again, as will be discussed later in this chapter, this is a marker for emotional volatility. So, based on the ClinicalQ EEG assessment, the clinician considers several hypotheses: this child may be exposed to bullying; he may have difficulty in school because of the mild attention issue; and he is emotionally depressed because of his poor performance academically and exposure to bullying. Further, the emotionality markers suggest that this may be a child who is highly emotionally reactive and may cry very easily. Of course, with his hypersensitivity, he would be a prime target for a bully.

So, to summarize the results of the ClinicalQ EEG brain wave assessment, this child has a mild marker for an attention issue; he has a marker for exposure to severe emotional stressors; he is showing a marker for reactive depression that may be associated with some event, or circumstance, to which the child has been exposed; and he is emotionally reactive and therefore a likely target for a bully.

There are some other issues indicated by the red highlighted numbers in the ClinicalQ. At location O1, the Theta/Beta ratio is a bit low under eyes closed condition. This is associated with poor stress tolerance and likelihood of poor sleep architecture. The latter can be important for the retention of the information a child learns during the day. If rapid eye movement (REM) sleep is deficient, the brain does not have adequate time to do the filing of information. REM is also important for emotional processing and of particular concern when working with clients with significant emotional trauma. In addition, at location Fz, there is a mild elevation in Delta amplitude, a condition that can affect attention. This elevation is very mild and will likely reduce in amplitude coincident with neurotherapy focused on decreasing the Theta/Beta ratio. Finally, again at location Fz, there is a mild elevation in the HiBeta–Gamma/Beta ratio indicating elevated activity of the anterior cingulate gyrus (ACG). This can result in perseverative thought processes and may exacerbate this child's emotional reactivity in the sense that once started he has difficulty regaining composure and again making him an attractive target for bullying.

Family Dynamics

The Case of the Kelly Family

Mrs. Kelly brought in her two children, Jane who was 7 years of age and Martin who was 9 years of age, for treatment of what her family physician thought was attention deficit disorder for both children. Fortunately for Mrs. Kelly, her family physician was strongly opposed to medicating children for ADHD, unless absolutely necessary. It may well have been that this very vigilant physician was

ClinicalQ Summary

Cz	xΘ/β	RΘ/β	α↑%	α↓%	TA
	2.86	3.12	18.3	1.6	58.5

O1	α↑%	α↓%	EO	EC
	-2.0	NA	2.33	1.69

	Θ/β	Θ/α
F4	2.53	1.87
F3	2.98	1.91

F=F%	β	α	Θ
	11.6	10.2	4.9

Fz	Dz	Hβ/β	∑	L/H	Θ/β
	17.8	0.70	15.3	1.98	3.0

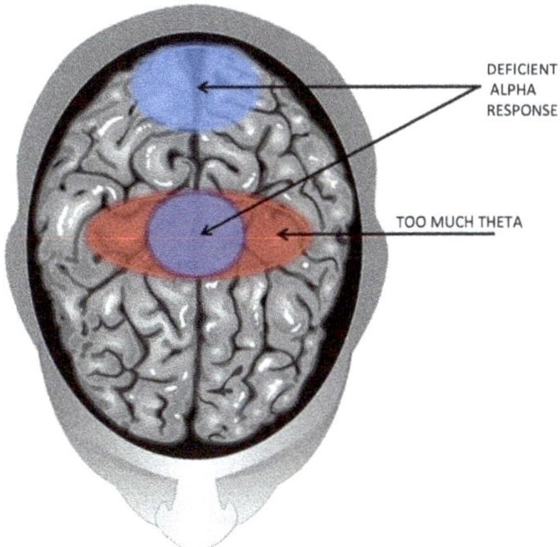

Fig. 3.23 ClinicalQ of 7-year-old Jane

suspicious that the problem with the children resided in problems with the family and that medicating this problem would be totally inappropriate.

The following are the data summaries for the ClinicalQ evaluations. The data critical to this discussion have been highlighted in red, and on the schematic brain diagrams, those areas have been highlighted. There are other areas in these summaries that are of clinical relevance but will not be addressed for the purposes of this discussion.

Figure 3.23 shows the initial intake clinical EEG assessment of Jane. Although Jane shows the EEG feature associated with ADHD (Theta/Beta ratio of 2.86 at location Cz), the feature of particular concern is the blunting of the Alpha response at both locations Cz and 01 (circled numbers—increase in Alpha should be at least 30 % at location Cz and at least 50 % at location O1). As the data show, the Alpha response was 18.3 % at Cz and slightly negative at location O1. These are the markers for exposure to severe emotional stress (Swingle 2013).

One EEG feature we often find with children who have severe attention problems is that they show the trauma marker. It is possible that the trauma is associated with fear of failure and humiliation in school associated with their attention and/or learning problems. However, whenever we see this pattern in children, we always determine if the child is being exposed to marked emotional stressors. This can be bullying, family strife, or some form of abuse. So in addition to neurotherapeutic treatment for the ADHD, we have to determine the cause of the Alpha blunting.

Mrs. Kelly had brought in both of her children at the same time for back-to-back appointments for the brain assessment. She was told by her physician that both children may have an ADHD problem.

ClinicalQ Summary

Cz	xθ/β	Rθ/β	α↑%	α↓%	TA
	2.98	2.63	0.0	NA	51.3
O1	α↑%	α↓%	EO	EC	
	39.6	2.4	2.29	2.39	
	θ/β	θ/α			
F4	2.89	2.01			
F3	2.56	1.91			
F=F%	β	α	θ		
	5.3	5.9	18.7		
Fz	Dz	Hβ/β	Σ	L/H	θ/β
	14.1	0.56	12.6	1.76	2.49

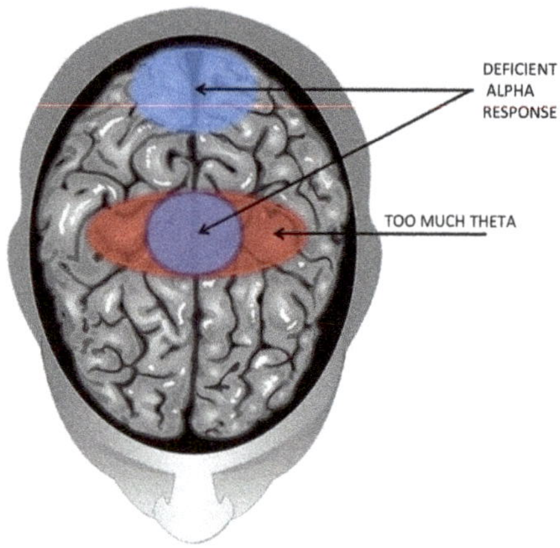

Fig. 3.24 ClinicalQ of 9-year-old Martin

As we can see in Fig. 3.24, Martin's EEG looked remarkably similar to Jane's. Both had the marker for ADHD (Theta/Beta ratio of 2.98 at location Cz). In addition, both had markers for exposure to severe emotional stressors. The Alpha blunting was in both locations Cz and O1 (Alpha response of zero at Cz and 39.6 % at O1), just as with Jane.

There are several important issues to consider here. First, given that we are seeing this marker with both children, it is possible that we are dealing with a genetic factor. Although Alpha blunting is highly correlated with exposure to severe emotional stressors (Swingle 2013), nonetheless, although rare, we do find it in situations in which there is no apparent present or historical exposure to emotional trauma.

The second issue is how we approach the mother in a manner that is not going to make her bolt from the therapeutic situation or make her severely distraught about her children's well-being. If there is no context in which this parent is aware of severe emotional stress, this kind of information can be clearly distressing. Parents immediately think about bullying, sexual predators, and other forms of abuse to which children might be exposed. It is extraordinarily important for the therapist to be able to deal with this situation in a manner that is rational and systematic.

The third issue is that healthcare providers have an obligation to report to the authorities any potential harm to a child. However, we have no direct evidence of this other than the EEG data. Recognizing that the parent may be the perpetrator, careful and prudent probing of the parent regarding the various conditions under which the emotional stress may occur, or have occurred, is required.

When I broached the subject of the children showing signs of being exposed to severe emotional stress, Mrs. Kelly broke down and admitted that there were severe problems in the family. According to Mrs. Kelly, her husband vacillated between severe depression and severe emotional abuse. He "flew off the handle" with minimal

ClinicalQ Summary

Cz	xΘ/β	RΘ/β	α↑%	α↓	TA
	2.79	2.68	-10.7	NA	30.4
O1	α↑%	α↓%	EO	EC	
	2.3%	4.9	1.69	1.55	
	Θ/β	Θ/α			
F4	0.80	1.49			
F3	1.51	1.93			
F=F%	β	α	Θ		
	191.1	38.9	9.8		
Fz	Dz	Hβ/β	Σ	L/H	Θ/β
	7.0	0.85	9.9	1.33	2.04

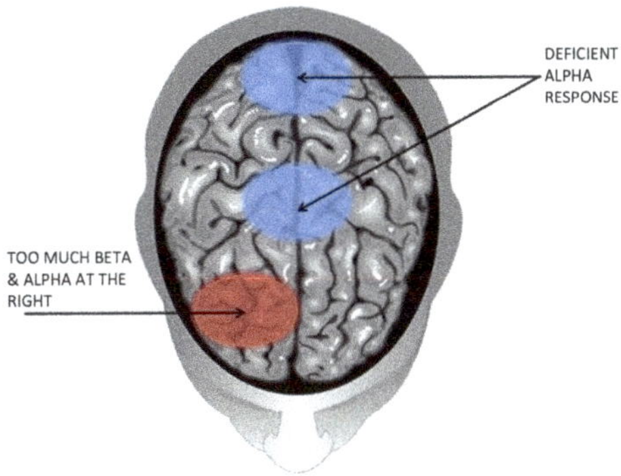

Fig. 3.25 Mrs. Kelly's ClinicalQ

provocation and was heavily medicated, and she felt that the children were severely disturbed by her husband's behavior. Mrs. Kelly agreed to let me measure her brain wave activity. Her ClinicalQ is shown in Fig. 3.25.

As can be seen in Fig. 3.25, Mrs. Kelly's EEG shows the marker for exposure to severe emotional stress, just as her children's. Her brain assessment also shows mild markers for problems with attention, again, just as her children, so she may be the source of the ADD markers that we find in her children. There are several other features of Mrs. Kelly's EEG that are important to note. The first is that she has a major marker for predisposition to depressed mood states; the amplitude of Beta activity is markedly greater in the right prefrontal cortex relative to the left. Whether the depression of Mrs. Kelly contributes to the family dynamic issue or whether it is the result of her exposure to the abusive behavior of her husband, nonetheless, children whose mother is severely depressed are profoundly more likely to have emotional behavior problems (Dawson et al. 1997; National Scientific Council on the Developing Child 2005; Seifer et al. 2001; Tronick and Reck 2009).

The second feature in Mrs. Kelly's ClinicalQ is that there is a marked elevation of Alpha amplitude in the right prefrontal cortex relative to the left. In children, we find this imbalance is often associated with oppositional and defiant behavior. In adult populations, we often find this disparity with individuals who are going through severe interpersonal problems such as marital discord, divorce, conflict in the workplace, and so forth.

It seems obvious that we are dealing with a family in crisis. Both of the children and Mrs. Kelly show markers for exposure to severe emotional stress (the blunted Alpha trauma markers). Mrs. Kelly shows a major marker for predisposition to depressed mood states, and on her intake self-report assessment, she describes herself as being one who falls into depression easily. Mrs. Kelly's description of her children's behavior, likewise, suggests that these children have some emotional difficulties. She describes Jane as easily upset, quick to anger, and unable to engage in cooperative play because she always must win. The latter condition, a child who must always win or they will refuse to play, is a cardinal marker for children who feel insecure and have negative self-regard. This is a characteristic often found with adopted children.

Mrs. Kelly describes Martin as being very anxious and unresponsive to others' feelings, and, importantly, she describes him as having behaviors associated with Internet addiction (addiction to video games). Internet addiction is an extraordinarily serious problem that is largely unrecognized by parents.

Although both children show the neurological pattern associated with common ADD, the central problems here are emotional and appear to result from family strife as opposed to being associated with attention deficit disorder. It is, of course, very likely that the ADD is contributing to the family strife. Such children require more assistance and more monitoring to complete their homework assignments, and they are usually experiencing difficulties in school, which puts further pressure on the family.

Our ability to diagnose the problem with the Kelly children as being primarily a problem with family strife testifies to the remarkable facility of the ClinicalQ EEG as a diagnostic instrument. Without any input from the parents, we were able to determine that family difficulties were giving rise to the problems that were affecting the children. Recall, the children were brought in for treatment because of difficulties in school. The assumption was that the children had some form of ADHD or other learning problem. This testifies to the accuracy of the EEG diagnostic procedure. Most importantly, however, it points out that other therapeutic strategies must be put in place to assist this family. Changing the neurology of the situation will be important, but it will be a minor component associated with the treatment of these children. It is extremely important to understand that family therapy and treatment of the parents will be equally as important as any kind of neurological work that we might do with the children.

We were most fortunate that Mr. Kelly not only recognized that he had serious problems but also recognized and acknowledged that his behavior was likely to be seriously affecting family functioning in a negative way. He further admitted that he thought his psychological problems were very likely interfering with the children's ability to perform efficiently in school. Mr. Kelly willingly came in for the ClinicalQ EEG assessment, the results of which are shown in Fig. 3.26.

Mr. Kelly described himself as follows: "I fly off the handle at minor problems. I'm anxious, depressed, and fatigued. I am on major medications including Wellbutrin, Cipralex, and Ativan that are not very effective. And I've been on other mixes of medications, all of which may have helped somewhat but eventually lost their effectiveness. I know that my behavior has seriously affected my marriage, my children, and my wife."

Although this situation is severe and complex, I am really tempted to take out the "cured" stamp at this point! Whenever one has clients who are willing to present themselves for treatment, are open and candid about their problems, and their potential detrimental influence on other individuals, the prognosis is extraordinarily good for a favorable outcome. We will have challenges in dealing with this situation, of

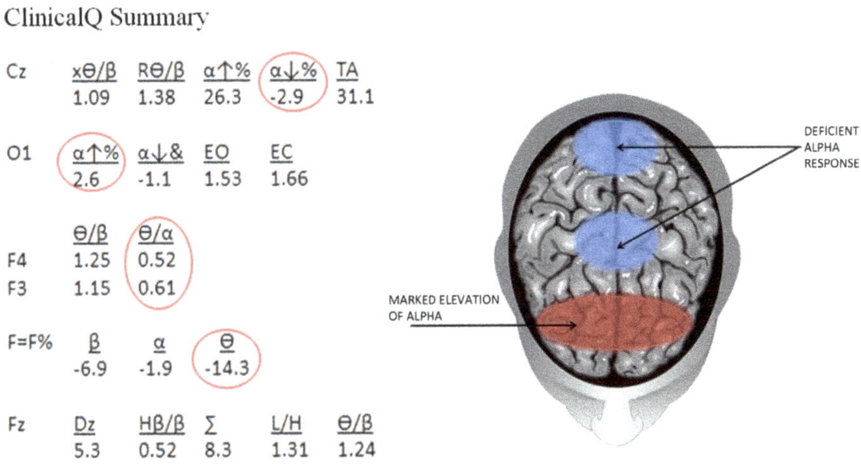

Fig. 3.26 Mr. Kelly's ClinicalQ

course. The challenges are not only neurological but behavioral in nature. Martin, for example, has developed a dependency on video games. This provides an escape and stimulation for this child, and it will be very difficult to wean him from this addictive behavior.

Mr. Kelly has a long history of dysregulated behavior and a long history of being medicated. Titrating him off the medications will also be a challenge. Nonetheless, given the data that we have on the neurological condition of each family member and the willingness of both parents to be candid about their condition and enthusiastic about presenting themselves for treatment, the prognosis bodes well for positive outcome.

Mr. Kelly's ClinicalQ indicated a number of anomalies that are interacting and exacerbating each other. That is, they are synergic in a negative sense. Mr. Kelly does not have the marker for the form of ADHD that the children show and, to some extent, Mrs. Kelly also. That form of ADHD is characterized by elevated slow frequency, primarily over the central part of the brain.

However, Mr. Kelly has an ADHD condition and a particularly nasty form, at that. He has marked elevation of Alpha amplitude in the front part of the brain (locations F3 and F4). The high frontal Alpha form of ADHD is characterized by problems with planning, organizing, sequencing, and following through on things (Swingle 2008). However, more importantly in this case is that high amplitude frontal Alpha is associated with emotional dysregulation. These individuals can have marked emotional volatility, problems with emotional impulse control, and difficulty sustaining emotional stability. Clients with this neurological condition are often diagnosed with bipolar disorder, personality disorder, and anxiety disorders in addition to ADHD.

Mr. Kelly also has a mild marker for depressed mood states in which the amplitude of slow-frequency Theta is greater in the left front part of the brain as opposed to the right. The predisposition to depression involves a number of conditions that result in the right prefrontal cortex being more active (aroused) than the left. Slow-frequency (Theta) amplitude was greater in the left relative to the right in Mr. Kelly's situation. When slow-frequency amplitude is greater in the left relative to the right, then the right frontal cortex will be more active than the left, a cardinal marker for depression.

Mr. Kelly has a few other situations that are giving rise to some difficulty. There is a deficiency of slow-frequency amplitude relative to fast-frequency amplitude (the Theta/Beta ratio) in the occipital region of the brain. Low ratio of the strength of Theta relative to Beta is associated with poor stress tolerance, predisposition to anxiety, sleep quality problems, and fatigue and often leads to self-medicating behavior such as excessive use of alcohol or prescription medications. Mr. Kelly's description of himself included many of the above. He described himself as "flying off the handle" at minor provocation, being anxious, depressed, and fatigued. Although individuals with low Theta/Beta ratios in the occipital region of the brain have a predisposition for self-medicating behavior, Mr. Kelly denied that he had any difficulty with alcohol. His wife substantiated this. He did comment, however, that he had a very long history of use of prescription medications.

Finally, we note that Mr. Kelly also has the marker for exposure to severe emotional stress. It is not an uncommon finding that the individual whose behavior is the fundamental cause of strife in the family also shows a marker for emotional trauma. It is difficult to know whether Mr. Kelly's trauma markers are associated with his present situation (family in turmoil) or whether this is an historical condition. Mr. Kelly's emotional difficulties may be associated not only with neurological conditions but also with the fact that he had been exposed to severe emotional trauma earlier in his life. Mr. Kelly did admit that he came from an extraordinarily violent household. During his early childhood, he lived in a constant state of fear and anxiety. Hence, it is not unlikely that Mr. Kelly's trauma markers are associated with childhood exposure to severe stress, whereas the markers we find in the brain assessments of the children and Mrs. Kelly reflect strife within the family, caused largely by Mr. Kelly's behavior.

It is also important to note that Mrs. Kelly has a major marker for depression and admits to severe depression episodes. Children of severely depressed parents, mothers in particular, are prone to serious emotional and cognitive problems. One might question if the cause of the family's turmoil is primarily Mrs. Kelly's depression exacerbated by Mr. Kelly's predisposition to dysregulated emotionality. These speculations are largely academic in that the treatment of the Kelly family is guided by the neurological conditions identified by the ClinicalQ and importantly with supportive family therapy to resolve the emotional distress and provide guidance for effective parenting. Reducing the emotional dysregulation of Mr. Kelly and the depression of Mrs. Kelly will likely resolve many of the issues affecting this family. And given the openness and willingness to receive treatment demonstrated by these parents, the prognosis is good.

Left-Handed Clients

With left-handed clients, the concern is the frontal-imbalance markers. There are certainly differences in brain laterality as has been documented, but are the emotional markers found for right-handed clients valid for left-handed clients as well? The data indicate no important differences for non-lateralized markers such as those at Cz, Fz, and O1. The evidence is quite clear that depression is associated with a hyperactive right hemisphere, and there is evidence indicating that such imbalances are associated with processing negative emotions and pessimistic thoughts. The extent to which these generalizations apply to left-handed clients is not clear. The data indicate that relative to the ClinicalQ assessment, the clinician is best advised to focus treatment on modulating any departures from the clinical database, independent of the degree of consistency with client descriptions of presenting complaints.

From the database of 110 left-handed and 732 right-handed adult clients, those whose ClinicalQ contained at least one marker for right frontal elevated activity, relative to the left, were selected. There were no significant differences between these groups in terms of ratings on the "I am depressed" questionnaire item. Analyzed in terms of the degree of imbalance associated with self-ratings of severe depression, left-handers had significantly less Beta imbalance ($t=2.17$, $p<0.03$, $df=310$) and overall lower Beta amplitudes in the right frontal cortex ($t=2.30$, $p<0.03$, $df=312$) but no significant differences in Beta amplitude in the left frontal cortex ($t=0.98$, *ns*). There were no significant differences between any of the other amplitude balance ratios based on the ratings of severity of depression or conversely ratings based on magnitude of the EEG amplitude imbalances.

Differences were found for clients with greater left frontal Beta amplitude imbalance. Selecting clients with left Beta amplitude that was at least 20 % greater in the left relative to the right frontal cortex, left-handed clients were more likely to rate themselves as depressed ($z=2.81$, $p<0.01$, $N=40$), anxious ($z=2.16$, $p<0.03$, $N=40$), easily frightened ($z=3.04$, $p<0.003$, $N=40$), and having sleep problems ($z=2.10$, $p<0.04$, $N=40$). All of these differences may be associated with anxiety rather than depression.

These subtleties are important because it alters the probing process during the initial intake session. The imbalances may have different implications although for the most part the differences between right- and left-handed clients are rather minor. The most important distinction is that the cardinal depression marker for right-handed clients (Beta elevated in the right relative to the left) is not as reliable for the left-handed person who may report anxiety rather than depression with this imbalance.

Seniors

Although the focus of this book is on neurotherapeutic treatment of brain functioning, when working with seniors, it is important to assess some vulnerabilities unique to this population. These conditions include exercise, sleep, diet, and purpose in life. The evidence is quite clear that exercise can be critical for the well-being of the elderly, so in addition to neurotherapy, simple devices like pedometers can be very effective for improving common complaints of health, fatigue, emotional state, and cognitive declines.

In a 2012 article in the journal *Neurobiology of Aging* (Fiocco et al. 2012), it was pointed out that a sure recipe for cognitive decline is salt and inactivity. In a 3-year study of more than 1,200 older adults with normal cognitive function at outset, researchers found that a high intake of sodium combined with low levels of physical activity was associated with a decline in global cognitive functioning. The authors go on to say that exercise may help immunize the brain against some of the adverse effects of higher sodium intake.

Katzmarzyk and Lee (2012) report that the relative risk for all-cause mortality was about 45 % higher for individuals sitting more than 6 h per day compared with those who sat less than 3 h per day. Further, watching TV for less than 2 h per day increases life expectancy by about 1.4 years. Research on college graduates average age 37 years found that the risk of death was twofold higher for participants who reported watching three or more hours of TV a day compared to those watching one or less hours (Basterra-Gortari et al. 2014).

It is also important to keep in mind that sitting for 6 h per day does not only implicate those who are sitting watching TV: It is unwise to sit for long periods of time. The recommendations are quite straightforward—one should get up about every hour and walk around for 5 min.

Walking actually affects subcortical structures in the brain. Colcombe et al. (2006) took a sample of 120 older adults without dementia who had been sedentary for the previous 6 months and gave a portion of them a walking regime. Those who were given the walking regimen showed about a 2 % increase in hippocampal volume compared with a contrast condition, where there was about a 1.5 % decrease.

A 7-year follow-up in a study of 2,340 seniors (mean age 74) found that deaths among slow walkers were almost three times greater than among fast walkers (>150 ft./min) (Odden et al. 2012). In another study (Bridenbaugh and Kressiq 2013), with a group of 1,153 older men (mean age 77), it was found that cognitive impairment progressed as walking gait slowed.

Haverman-Nies and De Groot (2003) conducted longitudinal research with about 2,200 seniors (70–75 years) exploring the effects of diet and activity on both vital and subjective well-being. Poor diet increased the occurrence of death by 1.2 in males and 1.3 in females. Inactivity increased the odds by 1.4 in males and 1.8 in females. Interestingly, inactive males were far more likely to rate their health as poor (odds ratio 2.8) as contrasted with females (odds ratio 0.8) even though inactive females had higher odds of death when inactive. These data again point to the major importance of activity for health with elderly clients.

Lifestyle improvements improve longevity even into old age (>75 years of age). Physical activities such as swimming, walking, or gymnastics were strongly related to longevity. Elderly who regularly engaged in these activities had a median age of death 2 years older than nonparticipants. Elderly who participated in one or more leisure activities and had a good social network had a median survival of 5.4 years greater than those with no leisure activities and poor social network (Rizzuto et al. 2012).

About 50 % of seniors report sleep problems, and those taking prescription sleep medications are at risk of slowing brain wave peak frequency which is associated with cognitive inefficiencies. From the ClinicalQ database, those rating themselves as forgetful had an Alpha Peak Frequency (APF) that, on average, was 4.4 % slower than those rating themselves as not forgetful ($t=2.34$, $p<0.03$, $df=41$). Alpha Peak Frequency is also related to client reports of poor health; those rating themselves high on the "I am physically unwell" item had an APF that was 7 % slower ($t=2.02$, $p<0.05$, $df=55$) than those rating themselves as a 1 on the question. Slowing of APF has been associated with age. Between the ages of 60 and 80, the APF declines by about 1 Hz; however, evidence suggests that these declines may be the result of neurological disease states experienced by the person and not age per se (Torres et al. 1983).

Adequate sleep architecture is as critical in old age as it is with younger people. Memory is directly related to adequate slow-wave sleep in the elderly (Oudiette et al. 2013). Oversleeping is associated with many health issues (Ohayon et al. 2013). Higher mortality rate (Kim et al. 2003), depression, cognitive inefficiencies, and many adverse health conditions are correlated with excessive sleep in elderly clients.

Finally, clients should be questioned about purposeful activities in their life. The data are quite clear about this matter. Boyle et al. (2009) used data from about 1,200 elders with an average age about 78 years. Self-rated purpose of life correlated negatively with self-rated depression (−0.32, $p<0.001$), as one might expect. However, controlling for self-rated depression and a number of other variables, purpose of life was associated with a substantially reduced risk of death; specifically, the hazard rate of a person with a high purpose of life score was about 57 % of the hazard rate for a person with a low (10th percentile) purpose of life score.

Prominent reasons that seniors seek neurotherapeutic treatment include depression, anxiety symptoms, health problems, and cognitive declines. Research has indicated that the prevalence of depression increases from a rate of 5 % at the age of 70 to approximately 13 % at the age of 85. A sample of seniors from 70 to 99 years of age was drawn from the ClinicalQ database to determine the efficacy of the cardinal Beta imbalance indicators for depression and anxiety. Frontal Beta imbalance, as a marker for depression, appears robust across age. Clients with Beta amplitude at least 15 % greater in the right rated themselves, on average, 70 % higher on the depression question as compared to clients with less than 10 % Beta imbalance ($t=2.35$, $p=0.03$, $df=17$). Seniors with left frontal elevated Beta amplitude of at least 15 % relative to those with less than 10 % imbalance rated themselves 50 % higher on the anxiety question ($t=2.39$, $p<0.04$, $df=10$) and 83.7 % higher on the "I feel tired and fatigued" question ($t=2.53$, $p<0.03$, $df=17$) and 52 % higher on the "I find it hard to concentrate" item ($t=2.24$, $p<0.04$, $df=16$). At location O1, seniors with Theta/Beta ratios below 1.0 rated themselves, on average, 38 % higher on the fatigue item relative to those with Theta/Beta ratios above 1.20 ($t=2.10$, $p<0.05$, $df=21$).

It appears as though some of the EEG markers for forgetfulness are not statistically sensitive to the variance in senior's reports of problems with retention and retrieval of information. This is likely the result of ceiling effects in the data since most seniors report such problems, and depression appears to be the more important condition associated with cognitive inefficiencies. This could be due to the emotional sequelae of depressed mood states such as lack of interest, motivation, and stamina, or it could be associated with the frontal neurological imbalances concomitant with depressed mood states. The imbalances could likely negatively affect efficient processing of information. In the clinical data set for seniors, only 3.4 % reported no problem with concentration as compared with 23.9 % of the adult database reporting no problems with concentration ($z=2.42$, $p<0.02$, $N=320$). The depression markers are sensitive to senior's reports of cognitive deficiencies as detailed above.

Conclusions

The data appear quite straightforward. Treat the neurological condition, not the label. Client self-reports are essential, of course, but they are not reliable indicators of how to proceed to treat the client. Here is where the one-size-fits-all franchisees have an advantage. Just like riding a stationary bicycle will have some general beneficial effects for virtually everyone, one size fits all will usually result in client reports of benefit. This is because of, not only, placebo effects, but also by stimulating brain wave contingencies, of whatever nature, the brain will generally show arousal and response to novelty.

The ClinicalQ offers the data for conducting the initial psychotherapy session in which the client's condition is not only validated, but more importantly their understanding of their condition is reorganized in neurological terms. The problematic areas have been identified for treatment. Important therapeutic concepts can be introduced for the client based on the neurological complications identified. Clients reporting "depression," for example, as discussed above, can understand that their emotional state is related to other conditions that make them feel hopeless and powerless.

People may feel tired and fatigued not because of sleep problems but because of depression or poor stress tolerance, or both. Clients may complain of problems with concentration when the problem is not ADD or aging but rather because of difficulties with being able to quiet the brain.

In general, as the above data indicate, the ClinicalQ is robust across many subgroupings of clients. Hence, the remarkable ranges can be used as reliable guides for clinical interventions as well as for developing the neurotherapeutic protocols.

Chapter 4
Neurofeedback

Although we will be discussing many treatment methodologies throughout this book, neurofeedback, or brain wave biofeedback, remains as the major "workhorse" in neurotherapy. As will be discussed in the next chapter, although other neurotherapeutic techniques such as braindriving, cranial stimulation, harmonic sounds, and the like are frequently used as adjunctive or even the major treatment for a client, neurofeedback remains as the procedure for stabilizing gains.

There are also many "stir-the-pot" procedures that have gained popularity and some reasonable data supporting efficacy for nudging the brain to reconfigure and reorganize. These procedures include z-score training, subcortical "region of interest" z-training, ultralow-frequency training, sLORETA z-training, and the like. Some of these procedures offer remarkable possibilities for expanding neurotherapy into regions of restructuring core emotional beliefs and hence more efficacious treatment for conditions such as eating disorders, disabling effects of severe emotional trauma, personality disorders, and the like. However, many of these procedures are marketed as one-size-fits-all, no-side-effects, and "anyone can do it" franchises. Thus, although I may start a client on braindriving and prescribe home use of one of the brain active harmonics, I will usually end regular treatment with at least a few sessions of brain wave biofeedback.

Neurofeedback is very straightforward. As we say, one simply "follows the map" for developing treatment protocols. What this refers to is doing neurofeedback over those brain sites that were identified as problematic in the initial brain assessment. Generally, neurotherapists have preferences in the manner in which they approach treatment in terms of which areas to treat first. In addition, there are decisions that one must make with respect to how to proceed with treatment. Does one stay with one problematic area until it comes within normative range or does one mix up the treatments, treating several different areas alternatively during treatment? Some areas are more difficult to treat and some brain wave ranges are more resistant to change.

In the present chapter, we will review some treatment considerations for each of the problematic areas covered in the ClinicalQ. The author's preferences for treatment sequences will be emphasized.

P.G. Swingle, *Adding Neurotherapy to Your Practice*,
DOI 10.1007/978-3-319-15527-2_4

Artifact

A serious problem with the measurement of any biological signal is that artifact is a particular problem with EEG recording. The EEG is affected by movement: movement of the client's body, movement of the facial and neck muscles, movement of the mouth and tongue, and, in particular, movement of the eyes. Some brain locations are more forgiving of some forms of movement; for example, eye movement is less likely to cause problems in the back of the head, whereas it is a huge problem with frontal recordings. Having the client keep their eyes closed can help, but even under eyes closed conditions, eye flutter is common and causes major corruption of the EEG recordings. For diagnostic purposes, one can shorten the measurement epoch and analyze only those epochs that seem relatively artifact-free. For treatment, most EEG feedback systems have an artifact rejection option, whereby if the recordings are outside some acceptable range, feedback is interrupted. The best option is an EEG feedback system that has a real-time EMG (electromyograph) which records muscle activity. The EMG signal is between 70 and 100 Hz, but usually one limits the artifact rejection to a narrower bandwidth. When the muscle activity is above threshold, the neurofeedback is interrupted (everything stops) until the EMG settles down, so one is not feeding back the muscle activity instead of EEG. Children can learn to move facial muscles to get rewards (movement of the game icons) instead of learning to modify brain wave activity. The real-time EMG is particularly useful when dealing with hyperactive children. Initially, the feedback game is set to train EMG, not EEG, so that the video game is responding to the muscle activity. The game proceeds (a child is rewarded) when he or she is still and not moving. Once the child quiets down, then the contingencies are shifted to EEG so that the game proceeds as a function of the child's EEG. This transition takes place without the child being aware of the change. The situation starts with quieting the child by making the contingency for reward a quieting of the body. Then, once the EMG levels decline, the contingency is changed by the neurotherapist "on the fly" to EEG with no interruption in the flow of the treatment session.

Some EEG feedback systems do not have real-time EMGs and rely on the total amplitude of all the EEG bandwidths as the artifact rejection system. Thus, when a client moves, the amplitude of all of the wave bands will increase. One sets the threshold for the total amplitude to say 100 μV, and when that threshold is passed, the neurofeedback is interrupted. This system is quite common in EEG systems, but in my opinion, it is not as good and certainly not as useful as real-time EMG artifact rejection.

The second source of artifact is an electromagnetically polluted environment. The source of the problem can be the 60 Hz of the electrical wiring. Many systems have a "notch" filter to exclude this source of artifact. Office machinery can also be a source of the EMF contamination, as well as any device that has an electrical motor. The latter sources can be particularly troublesome for the clinician because the problem tends to be intermittent in that it is only observable when the machinery is in use. Given that the machinery may be in some other office in the building, one cannot isolate the source of the problem. Cell phones have also been shown to cause problems with medical equipment (van Lieshout et al. 2007), and so I do not allow cell phones to be on in my office (they are annoying for other reasons as well).

The third source of corrupted data is static electricity. Not only can this be problematic in terms of the data, but static electricity can seriously damage the EEG equipment. Grounding is the best solution for static electricity. I make a habit of grounding myself before I touch the client and/or the equipment by touching a metal surface. In my clinic we also ground the client by putting a lead on the client's wrist and attaching it to the building ground (the casing of the 120 outlet is a building ground so attaching the lead to the screw holding the face plate on the outlet will work). Antistatic floor coverings and desk coverings that are likewise grounded to the building ground are also very helpful in reducing artifact. Having good electrode connections with low impedance is also very important in reducing artifact from EMF fields.

The fourth major source of corrupted data is the neurotherapist. The therapist is in the client's electrical field when working with the EEG. There are various levels to this. First, the location of the therapist can influence the EEG recordings. In a study of artifact problems associated with the movement and position of the therapist during neurofeedback (Swingle 1997), I found that there was a difference in the EEG amplitude of the various brain wave ranges, depending on where the clinician was standing during the recording. Recordings of the EEG at location Cz were obtained under two conditions: with the therapist directly behind the client and secondly with the therapist one meter to the client's left side. The differences in amplitudes were 2.3 % for Theta (*ns*), 13.1 % for Alpha ($t=2.95$, $df=6$, $p<0.05$), 7.3 % for SMR ($t=3.82$, $df=8$, $p<0.01$), 2.0 % for Beta (*ns*), 4.8 % for HiBeta (*ns*), and 14.1 % for EMG (70–90 Hz) ($t=2.42$, $df=8$, $p<0.05$).

Similarly, recordings were obtained for clients when they had their feet on an antistatic floor mat versus when they had at least one foot off the mat. Significant differences in amplitude were obtained for Theta, Alpha, and Beta at locations Cz and O1 (t values between 5.36 and 13.46, all p values <0.01). Thus, it is obvious that limiting the movement of the therapist, as well as the movement of the client, is important in obtaining clean EEG recordings and for a reliable feedback to occur. The general rule is "Whatever you do, ALWAYS do the same thing, and STAND STILL."

Treatment at Location Cz

Some clients come directly from heaven. Such is the case when one has a client with common ADD (CADD) as the only problem. Further, if this client is a female child of 8 years of age, or so, and comes from a loving, intact family whose love for this little girl is ABSOLUTELY independent of anything she does, then the neurotherapist can "bet the farm" that this child will be finished in 15–20 sessions and often considerably fewer. CADD (Swingle 2001) is the "non-attentive" form of ADD and is characterized by excessive Theta amplitude over the sensory motor cortex (Cz). The normative range for the Theta/Beta ratio in this region is below about 2.20, a bit higher for younger children. If the ratio is very high, such as above 3 or so, then we start seeing the hyperactivity component of the ADHD. At the higher ratios, the child becomes more in need of stimulation and the hyperactivity is self-stimulation. It is difficult at times to appreciate that it is actually "painful" for a child with this condition to sit still.

The basic treatment for CADD is simply Theta suppress, Beta enhance at location Cz. Because of the simplicity of this condition, I rarely resort to braindriving procedures but rely almost exclusively on neurofeedback. I also prescribe the OMNI harmonic for home use provided that in the initial assessment, the harmonic reliably suppresses Theta amplitude. As an example, consider the case of Jenny: a wonderful little 8-year-old girl from a loving, intact family of responsible and sensible parents. This case is of particular interest because it took 20 sessions, where normally with a simple case of this nature I would have predicted less than 15 sessions. The data were shown in the last chapter in Fig. 3.15, and the reader will recall that the Theta/Beta ratio got worse for the first 15 sessions and then Jenny "got it" and the Theta/Beta ratio dropped and stayed under the clinical cutoff.

It is critical for the therapist to keep parents from being so focused on the numbers that they abort treatment or discourage the child. Fortunately, this family stayed the course and Jenny made marvelous progress with correlated improvements in her schoolwork. Her self-esteem also was markedly boosted, a common effect of correcting ADD.

If on the assessment the client shows a Theta/Beta ratio within the normative range but a large Theta/Beta ratio when cognitively challenged (e.g., reading, counting backward), then braindriving may be a more appropriate treatment methodology. With braindriving using visual stimulation, the client can be engaged in a cognitive task while Theta is being suppressed. This is a very effective treatment for this form of ADD, in which the client is within normative limits on average and only shows the excess Theta amplitude under cognitive challenge. After a few sessions of braindriving, the client may then benefit from straightforward Theta/Beta training at location Cz. Neurotherapy continues until the challenged EEG shows a Theta/Beta ratio within normative limits.

If the brain assessment shows a deficient Alpha response (less than 30 % increase in Alpha from eyes open to eyes closed), then one should do Alpha amplitude enhancement, with eyes open and eyes closed. Generally, one focuses more on the eyes closed condition so the neurotherapy session is split about 75 % eyes closed and 25 % eyes open. Because Alpha blunting can be related to emotional trauma, the therapist should be vigilant regarding any emotional reactions of the client. The increase in Alpha can release memories and marked emotional reactions. This is a major therapeutic opportunity to help the client deal with the trauma, and I usually suspend the neurotherapy at this point and proceed to helping the client with the processing of the traumatic content. I also prepare the client for the possibility of increased dream activity associated with the trauma and that they are likely to be more mindful of the emotional aspects of the trauma for a few days. I also tell them that the neurotherapy has precipitated the most powerful psychotherapy on the planet, for we have engaged the natural psychotherapeutic processes of dreaming and mindfulness. Clients will often relate that they have "finally" processed the emotional trauma. For example, one female client had been burdened with severe guilt feelings associated with sexual molestation by her stepfather when she was in her early teens. She had experienced orgasm during these episodes and thus felt that she had been in some way responsible for this "shameful" behavior. After the release of the Alpha (both at Cz and also at O1), she emotionally accepted the fact that she had been "raped" and subsequently experienced pronounced emotional relief.

With children and especially those diagnosed with an autistic spectrum disorder, when the intake assessment shows a "hot midline," one should avoid starting treatment with Theta/Beta training at location Cz. The hot midline is when the HiBeta–Gamma/Beta ratio is much above 0.55 or when the summation of these two brain wave bands is above about 16. The reason one avoids the midline in these cases is because there is a possibility of exacerbating problems associated with the anterior cingulate gyrus if one increased the amplitude of Beta in that region. There have been several reports at conferences of cases of exactly this problem when Theta/Beta training was done over Cz with an autistic child. Hence, in the case of hot midline, one would usually decrease Beta and Gamma in that location before starting Theta inhibition.

Treatment at Location O1

Many neurotherapists avoid training in the parietal and occipital regions of the brain, particularly the occipital. The reason many avoid this area is because there is a significant potential for emotional abreaction and marked distress associated with the emergence of emotionally traumatic content. Therapists, who feel uncomfortable with working with distraught clients or those who feel unqualified, will avoid these areas and/or keep sessions brief and terminate at first hint of an emotional response. Those are the qualified therapists. Unfortunately, we have some unqualified therapists who do not have sufficient training and expertise to realize that they should avoid treating these areas. Fortunately, the one-size-fits-all franchises generally do not direct the often poorly qualified franchisees to train in the occipital areas.

On the other hand, for those qualified neurotherapists who treat emotional trauma, severe anxiety conditions, and addictions, treatment/training in the occipital region can be hugely beneficial to the client. "Releasing" the Alpha response and increasing the amplitude of Theta brain wave activity usually elicit strong emotional reactions in clients with significant emotional trauma histories. As pointed out in the section on symptoms associated with remarkable ranges at location O1, above, when the Theta/Beta ratio is much below 1.80, the client has problems finding peace in their head. When the Alpha response is weak or absent, then the client likely has a significant emotional trauma history. When training at location O1, increasing the Theta/Beta ratio will have the effect of quieting the mind. A by-product of this quieting for the client with trauma is emotional abreaction, which can vary in intensity and include any or all of the sensory modalities.

There are several suggested guidelines for treatment in the occipital areas. Because one is attempting to quiet the client, many clinicians start training with a few sessions of peripheral biofeedback such as thermal (e.g., hand-warming) or electromyographic (EMG) to reduce muscle tension.

I have found that it is helpful to do an autonomic nervous system stress assessment to determine the exact peripheral system that would be most efficient for relaxing the client. Thus, for clients who show most responsiveness in the EMG, I would prescribe a home muscle relaxation exercise such as progressive muscle relaxation and a few EMG biofeedback sessions on the frontalis muscles (forehead) prior to commencing the neurofeedback. For clients who show most responsiveness in the thermal system, I would prescribe a home hand-warming exercise and a few sessions of hand-warming biofeedback. For those who respond with accelerated heart rate, I prescribe heart rate autogenic exercises for home use and heart rate biofeedback. For those who respond with increased electrodermal activity, I prescribe breathing exercises for home use and would do some electrodermal biofeedback training often before starting a neurotherapy session.

Heart rate variability (HRV) training has been shown to increase the amplitude of the sensory motor rhythm (13–15 Hz; SMR) (Reid and Nihon 2011; Reid et al. 2013). As will be discussed in a later chapter, HRV can be used prior to a neurotherapy session to facilitate relaxation and concentration.

One can proceed directly to neurofeedback and many neurotherapists prefer to do just that. One can start training with increasing Alpha amplitude, eyes closed at location Pz. This location is easier to train and if the client is told to simply relax and visualize a sailing ship going over the horizon, one usually sees an increase in the amplitude of Alpha. When I start directly with neurofeedback, in addition to increasing Alpha in office, I usually prescribe the Mozart harmonic, described in the next chapter, for home use. This harmonic has the effect of increasing the Alpha amplitude and facilitates the in-office treatments. After the client gains some facility at increasing Alpha, one usually sees that Theta amplitude starts to increase. At that time I generally switch the electrode to position O1 and proceed with a few more Alpha increase neurofeedback sessions. When Theta starts to increase in amplitude, the contingency is switched to include Theta and then exclusively Theta. When the Theta amplitude finally exceeds the Alpha amplitude, one usually sees an emotional reaction.

A low Theta/Beta ratio in the occipital region can also be the result of excessive Beta amplitude. In this case one usually does Beta suppress neurotherapy or Beta suppress, Theta enhance. There are some qualitative differences, I have observed, between clients who present with excess Beta amplitude and those who have a deficiency in Theta amplitude. Clients who have similar Theta/Beta ratios can appear quite different when one is Beta excessive as opposed to Theta deficient. The Beta excessive, I find, appears more noticeably agitated. Both conditions are correctable with neurotherapy, but of course, one is altering different aspects of the ratio, either

Beta or Theta or perhaps both. I have found that enhancing Theta responds more quickly than suppressing Beta amplitude.

Braindriving, to be covered in the next chapter, is particularly useful for the treatment of conditions in the occipital region. Braindriving can often bring a client very rapidly to near normative ranges and potentiate significant emotional reactions in a few sessions. This emotional content then can be a focal point for other therapy to help the client process trauma. Although the braindriving can markedly accelerate treatment, I always return to straightforward neurofeedback to stabilize the Theta/Beta ratio.

A pattern that is quite commonly observed with the more aggressive treatments for emotional trauma is rather like the reverse of the Theta crossover Alpha dynamic associated with emotional abreaction. Often, the client will show a marked increase in Theta amplitude and then a rapid increase in Alpha followed by a Theta amplitude decline. This pattern is associated with the clients' experiential reports of a sensation of calming followed by troubling emotional thoughts or memories (coincident with the rise in Alpha amplitude).

For clients without significant trauma history, the normalization of the Theta/Beta ratio in the occipital region usually results in reports of being more relaxed, calmer, better able to concentrate, more global appreciation of concepts, better sleep, more emotional grounding, better stress tolerance, more rested feelings, more positive attitudes, and less behavioral urgency (e.g., reduced impatience, reduced appetitive urges).

Generally, starting treatment with improving the occipital regions is a good initial treatment. Clients usually report favorable effects very rapidly in terms of feeling more relaxed and at peace. The credibility of treatment efficaciousness is thereby again enhanced, having been strongly implanted with the accuracy of the interpretive ClinicalQ.

Related treatments for calming include reducing the Theta/SMR ratio over locations C3, Cz, and C4. This treatment, Theta suppress, SMR enhance is, of course, the treatment for seizure disorders and has the effect of calming. When a client has a deficiency in the Theta/Beta ratio in the occipital region and also complains of some pain condition, such as migraine headaches, I often combine treatment at O1 with decreasing the Theta/SMR ratio at C4. This combination is very effective for the anxious client with headaches.

Another very effective treatment for postural and motor difficulties is Margaret Ayers' protocol at locations just below O1 and O2. The electrode placement is a bipolar montage at locations right under the occipital ridge just below O1 and O2. The protocol is to mildly inhibit 4–8 Hz and enhance 15–18 Hz. I often pair this treatment with the Theta/Beta enhance at location O1 or O2. Because of the proximity of the two treatment locations and the somewhat conflicting protocols (i.e., enhance Beta range and suppress Theta range brain wave amplitude at just below O1/O2, whereas the reverse is trained just a few millimeters away), I often alternate these treatments being guided of course by observed changes in the data and by the client's reports.

If one is experiencing difficulty with increasing the Theta/Beta ratio in the occipital regions, a useful procedure is to move the electrodes to P3 or P4 or to do a bipolar placement at O1 and O2. Often one will find that clients are better able to have success with the latter placements when the unipolar O1 or O2 is not being successful. Alternatively, one can use braindriving procedures (described in the next chapter) to potentiate the Alpha/Theta training and then return to the conventional neurofeedback to stabilize the gains.

Treatment at Locations F3 and F4

Although there are many disorders that are associated with various imbalances in the frontal cortex regions, treatment in these areas is very straightforward and often results in fast and important changes noted by the clients. Because imbalance is such an important issue in the client's well-being, treating excessive amplitude in a particular region must be done with great caution so as not to precipitate a problem by creating an imbalance. For example, high Theta/Beta ratios at F3 and F4 are associated with cognitive, attention, and learning inefficiencies and often some difficulties with fine motor coordination affecting writing and small object assembly. The treatment of this excess is to suppress Theta and/or to enhance Beta amplitude in each of the two frontal lobes. A bipolar placement at F3 and F4 can be used with a Theta inhibit Beta enhance protocol. The area to watch is usually the waveform that one is enhancing. Because the placement is bipolar, increasing the amplitude of a brain wave can have the effect of increasing the difference between the two electrode sites. The differential amplifier on the EEG feedback system is giving feedback on the difference between the two sites so one could be causing greater imbalances in the frontal regions. Imbalances are always potentially problematic, so I always keep a careful watch when using bipolar placements and discontinue this form of treatment if differences start to occur. In that case, I either switch back to unipolar placement and continue the training alternating between the two sites or use the very effective two-site braindriving procedure described in the next chapter.

Excessive Alpha amplitude in the frontal regions likewise should be treated with caution. This form of ADD responds more slowly to treatment than many other forms of ADD. In this case, I again will train down the Alpha using either bipolar or alternating unipolar electrode placements. Imbalances in Alpha amplitude in the frontal lobes are associated with several conditions including depression and oppositional and defiant behavior. Hence, one wants to be cautious when inhibiting Alpha amplitude to do so in such a way as to minimize any imbalances.

For depressed clients, one can generally improve their mood state by arousing the left frontal cortex by either increasing Beta amplitude in the left or decreasing Alpha or Theta amplitude in the left. Which of these alternatives the neurotherapist selects is based on the results of the ClinicalQ. When both Alpha and Theta have greater amplitude in the left, relative to the right, frontal cortex, then one may also downtrain Thalpha (3–9.5 Hz). In general, if the depression is reactive in nature, such as grieving over the death of a loved one, I do not downtrain the slow frequencies aggressively. The grievance process should be allowed to proceed unimpeded. This is precisely the mega-mistake physicians often make in prescribing antidepressants for persons engaged in a normal grieving process. What I certainly would train aggressively in such cases is an imbalance of Beta amplitude when the right is greater than the left, for this is a predisposing condition for depression. Correcting this predisposition does not interfere with the normal grieving process but gives the client some relief in that the predisposition to depressed mood states will not exacerbate the reactive depression.

If there is an excessive total amplitude (i.e., summation of the amplitudes of Theta, Alpha, and Beta at any site) in the frontal regions, rather than do the "squash" protocol (i.e., training down 3–25 Hz) at F3 or F4, I usually do this training at Cz. One is less likely to trigger any imbalance problems and one generally finds that as the total amplitude (TA) decreases at location Cz, there is a related decrease in this summated value at the frontal locations as well.

The use of the braindriving procedures described in the following chapter is very helpful for treating disparities in the frontal cortex. In addition, bilateral stimulation procedures such as EMDR and the SWEEP harmonics (also described in the next chapter) can be very effective in balancing the frontal lobes. For clients in distress associated with these imbalances, braindriving is the treatment of choice.

Training at Location Fz

The most critical issue associated with treatment at this location is to avoid activation if the center midline is "hot." If the HiBeta/Beta ratio is much above 0.55 or the summation of the amplitudes of these two brain wave bands is above 15, then avoid any Theta suppress or Beta increase at this location. If the frontal area is "hot," then behaviors associated with that location such as worrying, fretting, perseveration, and obsessive/compulsive behaviors can be exacerbated with arousal enhancing treatment protocols. Thus, a person with some obsessive/compulsive behaviors or the autistic child with perseverative behaviors may become more symptomatic if stimulating protocols are used.

When the summated amplitude of HiBeta–Gamma and Beta is greater than 15 and the client admits to excessive worrying and fretting, then the inhibit protocols are appropriate. Since one must also be concerned with the ratio of these two brain wave bands, inhibits should be designed so that the ratio of HiBeta–Gamma/Beta remains within the 0.45–0.55 normative range. Thus, one might inhibit HiBeta–Gamma or Beta or both to bring the summated value below 15 and the ratio around 0.50. Because of the artifact problem, treatment at this location is generally done with eyes closed. For autistic spectrum clients who may have problems keeping their eyes closed or have significant eye movement even with eyes closed, braindriving under eyes open conditions is an option. This protocol is described in the next chapter.

To correct the ratio, again one must consider whether the ratio is outside the normative range because of the HiBeta–Gamma or the Beta or both and train accordingly. I often downtrain the full range of 16 through 40 Hz for a few sessions and then downtrain the HiBeta–Gamma to keep the ratio around 0.50.

For very low ratios, well below 0.45, one trains up the HiBeta–Gamma to bring the ratio into the normative range. However, even with low ratios, it is not recommended that the ratio be increased unless the client admits to excessive passivity.

Excessive Delta amplitude, above 10 μV or so, does not usually occur in isolation, but generally one also finds excessive Theta amplitude in the frontal brain regions as well. Further, when one finds high frontal Delta, it is likely that the Delta is elevated in other brain areas as well. Pain, for example, is often associated with elevated Delta not only in the frontal regions but spread toward the back of the brain. Given that Delta is often associated with elevated Theta in the frontal regions, training Theta first may be most efficient since Delta may decline in amplitude coincident with Theta downtraining. Delta in the frontal regions is markedly affected by muscle artifact of the eyes and facial muscles. Children often learn quickly that they can have great fun moving their facial muscles to make the game icons stop and go. Unfortunately, under these conditions nothing much is happening with the Delta amplitude. It is for these conditions that a real-time EMG is very useful. One can set the contingencies so that muscle quiet is trained and once the child is quieted then switch to Delta feedback. Braindriving is also very effective for Delta downtraining.

Brain efficiency, at least in terms of the prevention of dementias and other age-related declines, can be measured in several ways. A common method is to measure the dominant frequency in the Alpha (8–12 Hz) range; the faster the peak frequency, the more efficient the brain. A second measure is the density of slow to fast Alpha. The amplitude of slow Alpha (8–9 Hz) divided by the amplitude of fast Alpha (11–12 Hz) gives the Alpha density ratio; the lower the ratio, the more efficient the brain. There are EEG feedback systems that can give a leading edge feedback. This form of neurofeedback gives feedback when the peak frequency of a particular brain wave band is increasing. For the leading edge feedback of Alpha, for example, the feedback tones would occur when the Alpha band peak frequency is increasing over the set threshold frequency. Thus, if the threshold were set for say 10.4 Hz, then feedback would occur for any peak frequency above that value. Some feedback is also analog so that the intensity or frequency of the tone increases the greater the distance of the measured frequency from the threshold frequency. For example, a peak frequency of 11.0 Hz would be louder or higher in pitch than a peak frequency of 10.8 Hz, but the sound would be on in both cases because the peak frequency is greater than the threshold frequency of 10.4 Hz.

Because Alpha Peak Frequency (APF) training with most manufacturers' software is, at present, based on average APF over a time period, the reward tones are not contingent on a response. An average is not an event. Hence, at present, the efficiency of these training protocols may be limited. An alternative method is to uptrain the high-frequency band and downtrain the lower-frequency band. Thus, as is my preference, I reward the 11–12-Hz amplitude and I inhibit the 8–9-Hz amplitude. In this protocol, the relative density of the faster Alpha activity is increased and the relative density of the slower Alpha is decreased. Training continues until the ratio of fast to slow drops below 1.50. I usually continue training to bring the ratio considerably below the 1.50 cutoff.

Summary

Neurofeedback training is very straightforward. It is objective and data driven. When one notes departures from some normative clinical value, then one trains to bring that activity within the normative range. The client is fully informed of the purpose of the training and understands that the purpose of the treatment is to modify the symptoms associated with the brain wave anomalies noted on the ClinicalQ. If the client is depressed because of an imbalance in Beta amplitude in the frontal cortex, then the client expects to be less depressed when the imbalance is corrected.

As a rule, I start from the back of the brain and move forward. At the back, deficiencies are associated with problems with mental quiet. Once this has been improved, as indicated by an increase in the Theta/Beta ratio, then the training is moved forward to correct anomalies in the frontal regions. If one is dealing with trauma, then after the Alpha is released in the occipital region, the Alpha is also released at Cz if it has not already corrected itself.

With ADD and ADHD children, on the other hand, I would generally correct the excess slow frequency at Cz and the frontal regions first and then proceed to correct other anomalies. Excessive frontal slow-frequency amplitude usually improves with improvements at the central locations.

For balancing frontal lobe amplitudes, in general, decrease the slow frequencies first and then move to the Beta frequencies. Beta uptraining is difficult and many neurotherapists maintain that Beta cannot be trained in the frontal regions. This is not so as one can train any brain wave either with volitional neurofeedback procedures or with some of the non-volitional procedures discussed in the next chapter. Often bipolar placement with downtraining the brain wave band (the so-called poor man's coherence training) can help with restoring balance in the frontal lobes.

Chapter 5
Potentiating Neurotherapy

Many neurotherapists provide clients with various adjunctive self-administered treatments to facilitate the therapeutic process. These adjunctive complementary treatments include relaxation exercises, self-hypnosis, energy psychology routines, lifestyle modification recommendations, subliminal affirmation devices, cranial microamperage stimulators, audiovisual stimulators, and therapeutic harmonics. The reason for prescribing these procedures, of course, is that they potentiate the therapeutic process.

I have been particularly interested in the use of therapeutic harmonics, and I have been doing research in this area for several decades. One such harmonic (OMNI) is a blend of several carrier frequencies providing a dominant 10 Hz overriding frequency that is embedded in a filtered pink noise at between –15 and –25 dB(C). The effect of the OMNI harmonic is that it suppresses EEG Theta (3–7 Hz) amplitude (Swingle 1996) and has been found to markedly accelerate the neurotherapeutic treatment of common attention deficit disorder (CADD) (Swingle 2001). The OMNI harmonic has been used by thousands of clients and is marketed by several companies. The data on this harmonic are very consistent. The suppressing effect is about the same with males and females [provided the sound pressure levels are presented at gender-specific levels; see Swingle (1992)], but differs with age. For clients over 18, the suppression of Theta amplitude is about 30 %, whereas for young children the suppression is about 15 %.

It is not surprising that sound influences brain activity and we certainly have a lot of research that substantiates that view. My own research has identified a number of harmonic blends that have specific effects on the EEG. Such effects include reducing Beta amplitude, increasing Theta amplitude, balancing frontal lobe brain activity, increasing the SMR, increasing the density of fast Alpha (11–12 Hz) relative to slow Alpha (8–9 Hz), increasing Alpha amplitude during eyes closed periods, suppressing high-frequency (28–40 Hz) amplitude, enhancing sleep quality, as well as decreasing Theta amplitude over Cz. These harmonics can be very useful as adjunctive treatments to facilitate, potentiate, and stabilize neurotherapy.

P.G. Swingle, *Adding Neurotherapy to Your Practice*,
DOI 10.1007/978-3-319-15527-2_5

When working with subtle energy such as subliminal harmonics, it is important to prepare the stimuli so that they are within the effective range. In the case of sound, the effective range is very specific and narrow [techniques for preparing such materials are described in Swingle (1992)]. If the sound is too close to supraliminal levels, the information is not processed. This "gray zone" is found not only with sound but with other modalities as well (Gary Schwartz, personal communication, reported this gray zone with olfaction, and Len Ochs, personal communication, reported this for visual stimulation). This suggests two independent processing systems for information above and below perceptual thresholds and, importantly, an energy level zone in which the information is not processed efficiently in either system.

The second finding suggesting that subtle energy may be processed differently from more potent stimulation is that identical stimuli produce different effects supraliminally versus subliminally. For example, when presented at 15 dB(C) below ambient, a 10-Hz harmonic increases heart rate, whereas a 25-Hz harmonic at the same intensity reduces heart rate, which is the opposite of what one would expect with a supraliminal presentation of these same frequencies (Ohatrian et al. 1960; Swingle 1993).

We proceed now to reviewing the research on the harmonics that influence EEG activity. These harmonics can be used for braindriving or they can be used statically by clients in their home environments. Following the section on the harmonics, protocols for driving EEG activity will be reviewed.

Treatment Harmonics All of the harmonics described in this section can be prepared by the clinician following the directions in the book *Subliminal Treatment Procedures: A Clinician's Guide* (Swingle 1992a, b) and in articles describing the use and preparation of specific harmonics (Swingle 1996, 2001). The essential features of all of the harmonics to be described below are that they are embedded in filtered pink noise with a 50-dB roll-off at 1,000 Hz. The carrier frequency for the blended sounds is 300 Hz, so, for example, the Theta-suppressing OMNI harmonic has a beat frequency of 10 Hz created by blending 300 Hz with 310 Hz. All of the beat frequencies are based on the 300 Hz carrier frequency. The beat frequency harmonics are embedded at between 15 and 25 dB below the embedding filtered noise. Research described in Swingle (1992a, b) found that males and females respond optimally at different subthreshold amplitudes. Females are more affected by sounds at minus 25 dB and males respond more to sounds at 15 dB below the embedding pink noise. Clinicians should note that the effect of beat frequencies presented below threshold are often very different from what one would expect with the same blend presented above hearing threshold. The Theta-suppressing OMNI harmonic, for example, contains a 10-Hz beat frequency, yet it suppresses Theta amplitude. Research further has shown that even beat frequencies in the Theta range (i.e., 5 Hz) suppress Theta amplitude when presented at sound levels well below hearing thresholds (Swingle 1996).

For clinicians who do not wish to prepare their own harmonics, CDs and sound files downloadable from the web are available from a number of suppliers including soundhealthproducts.com, futurehealth.org, toolsforwellness.com, prpress.com, and mindalive.com. In addition the two major manufacturers of clinical EEG neurofeedback systems (Thought Technology and BrainMaster) have software suites that provide a limited number of the harmonics described in this chapter. There are also many companies that supply frequency sound generators for clinicians who wish to develop their own sound stimuli.

As the reader may recall from Chapter two, it was recommended that as part of the ClinicalQ, the clinician should test a harmonic to determine the precise effect on the client's brain wave activity. Routinely, the Theta-suppressing harmonic is tested at location Cz, but one could, of course, test any of the harmonics during the rapid intake procedure. The benefit of this procedure is to demonstrate convincingly to the client that the harmonic has a clear and demonstrable effect on brain activity so when prescribed by the clinician the effectiveness has been established. In other words, there is no guesswork or experimentation with different harmonics since one can establish that the harmonic has the desired effect. This is in striking contrast, of course, to the traditional methods of treatment. Traditionally, the client would expect a physician, for example, to prescribe a medication for the client to try, and if it works, fine; if not, another is tried.

The harmonics described in the following section include OMNI, SERENE, and SWEEP. The OMNI family of harmonics is used to suppress the amplitude of Theta (3–7 Hz). The SERENE harmonics are used to increase Theta amplitude, decrease Beta amplitude, and decrease 28–40-Hz amplitude. The SWEEP harmonic was designed for use in bilateral stimulation applications such as variants of rapid eye movement desensitization (EMDR). It was found that the SWEEP harmonic has the effect of balancing brain wave amplitude in the frontal lobes. Hence, SWEEP was found to be very effective in braindriving applications. There are many other harmonics that are used for specific purposes. However, the basic harmonics that are most often used in braindriving applications and prescribed for home use are OMNI, SERENE, and SWEEP. The discussion below, therefore, is limited to these basic harmonics.

OMNI The essential feature of this harmonic is that a 10 Hz beat frequency is embedded in filtered pink noise. This harmonic has been heavily researched for over a decade. The important use of this harmonic is to suppress the amplitude of Theta and to increase the density of fast Alpha (11–12 Hz) relative to slow Alpha (8–9 Hz). The latter can also be indicated by an increase in the dominant frequency of Alpha related to exposure to the OMNI harmonic. Theta suppression averages about 15 %, is somewhat higher for females than males, and is positively correlated with age, that is, more suppression for older clients (Swingle 1994). Home use of the OMNI harmonic reduces Theta amplitude as measured at location Cz by about one percent per week over an 8-week test period (Dupont and Swingle 1996).

The OMNI harmonic is used for braindriving to suppress the slow-frequency EEG amplitude or to increase the relative density of fast Alpha. These harmonics are also prescribed for home use to enhance focus and attention such as for children with ADD when they are doing school homework. The harmonics are also prescribed to facilitate neurotherapy and to sustain the gains made during neurotherapy treatments.

Budzynski (1995) tested the OMNI harmonic and found that it also appears to increase 14-Hz amplitude over the sensory motor cortex. Since 14-Hz training has been found to be helpful in the treatment of migraine headache, OMNI can be prescribed for home use to increase and/or sustain SMR brain wave amplitude. Swingle (1996) reports that a client with migraine headache did report modest relief from pain with home use of OMNI.

Theta suppression correlates with total amplitude (TA), which is the sum of the amplitudes of Theta, Alpha, and Beta at location CZ ($r=0.31$, $p<0.001$, $N=914$). But OMNI Theta suppression does not correlate above $r=0.30$ with any other ClinicalQ EEG measures at any other of the ClinicalQ sites.

SERENE The SERENE harmonic reduces heart rate and increases slow-frequency brain wave amplitude at several locations including the occipital and parietal sites. Heart rate reductions for a nonclinical population of college students ranged from 1.2 % to 3.5 %, and for a clinical population, the reductions averaged about 3 % after a 1-min exposure to the SERENE harmonic (Swingle 1992a, b).

The essential feature of the SERENE harmonic is a blend of frequencies that give a beat frequency of 25 Hz. As with the OMNI harmonic, the carrier frequency for SERENE is 300 Hz and the blended tone is 325 Hz. The sound pressure level modulates between −15 dB(C) and −25 dB(C) to present the harmonic in the ranges most appropriate for both males and females (Swingle 1992a, b).

One of the major uses for the SERENE harmonic is to increase the amplitude of Theta brain waves in the occipital regions of the brain. Twenty-one clients drawn from our database had exposure to the SERENE harmonic during the intake assessment ClinicalQ. The exposure was for 45 s with the EEG electrode over site O1. The average percent change in Theta amplitude was 26.3 % ($SD=22.8$, $t=5.31$, $p<0.001$, $N=21$). Of the total sample, 4.3 % of the clients did not respond to the harmonic with an increase in Theta amplitude.

Another sample of 39 clients was exposed to the SERENE harmonic, while the HiBeta–Gamma brain waves were being measured at location Fz. The SERENE harmonic was presented for 30 s. The average decrease in the amplitude of this brain wave range was 15.4 % ($SD=8.9$, $t=11.0$, $p<0.001$, $N=39$). Of the 39 clients, 13.3 % did not show any decrease in HiBeta–Gamma amplitude.

SERENE has also been found to be effective to reduce frontal Beta as measured at location Fz. Fifty-three clients were exposed to the SERENE harmonic for 45 s during the intake ClinicalQ. Of the 53 clients, 18.9 % did not respond to the SERENE harmonic. Of the 43 who did respond, the average suppression in Beta amplitude was 12.3 % ($t=9.84$, $SD=8.2$, $p<0.001$, $N=43$).

Because the harmonic has the effect of both reducing the amplitude of brain waves in the 16–40-Hz range and increasing the amplitude of Theta in the occipital region of the brain, SERENE is used for many purposes including relaxation, sleep quality improvement, reduction of obsessive and compulsive thoughts and behaviors, and reduction of fretting.

SWEEP The harmonic used in SWEEP is a blend of five tones in the range of 300 Hz. Because of the multiple tones, SWEEP generates many beat frequencies and a complex harmonic. The "sweep" aspect of the harmonic is that it moves back and forth between the right and the left headset earphone at an excursion rate of 4.5 s. There is a brief pause at each extreme. This harmonic has been used by many certified EMDR clinicians who find it effective as a form of bilateral stimulation used in client treatment. In particular, these clinicians have reported that SWEEP is particularly useful for the treatment of clients who have a history of traumatic stress.

When SWEEP is used to facilitate the processing of traumatic content, the client is instructed to simply close their eyes and allow any emotional content to emerge. Various prompts are provided to help the client move through the fear and marked anxiety that usually accompany the emergence of traumatic memories. The emergence of traumatic memories is generally accompanied by a marked and rapid increase in Theta amplitude. One such example was a young woman of 35 who had been sexually molested as a young child by a female family friend. When the traumatic memory emerged, the Theta amplitude increased by 32.3 % and stayed elevated for about 8 min. The Alpha and Beta amplitudes declined slightly during that same period. The client's heart rate also increased during that time by about 39 %.

Although SWEEP is often prescribed for home use, in the present context the use of SWEEP is to balance the brain wave amplitudes between the two frontal lobes. SWEEP is often used in conjunction with braindriving of Theta amplitude in the occipital areas of the brain to facilitate frontal balancing while the braindriving is calming the client. One example is a 17-year-old client with an autistic spectrum disorder. Prior to exposure to SWEEP, the imbalances in brain wave amplitude in the frontal lobes were 28.2 % for Theta, 33.0 % for Alpha, and 18.7 % for Beta, all greater in the right relative to the left. Each of these imbalances exceeds the ClinicalQ threshold for clinical significance. After exposure to SWEEP, the imbalance percentages were 5.8 %, 21.6 %, and 13.3 % for Theta, Alpha, and Beta, respectively. Note that two of these differences are below the clinical threshold after treatment and the percent change ranged from 28.9 % for Beta, 34.5 % for Alpha, and 79.4 % for Theta.

SWEEP can be particularly effective for the rapid treatment of some forms of depression for those clients who present themselves for treatment early in the depression state. For those forms of depression in which there is an imbalance in the Theta amplitude in the frontal cortex, with the left (F3) having 15 % or greater higher amplitude than the right (F4), SWEEP followed by Theta downtraining neurofeedback at location F3 can be particularly effective. Often, these clients report significant relief after a single session. An example of the latter was a client who sought treatment for his depression within 1 month of his becoming aware of the problem. He was not on any medication so one would expect rapid response to any neurotherapeutic treatment. His form of depression was the imbalance of the Theta amplitude in the frontal cortex, as described above, in addition to some other markers for predisposition to depressed mood states. His Theta amplitude imbalance was 13.8 %, the Alpha imbalance was 8.6 %, and the Theta/Beta ratio imbalance was 21.5 %, all with the left (F3) greater than the right (F4). The treatment was a 15-min exposure to the SWEEP harmonic followed by Theta downtraining neurofeedback at location F3. After the 15-min exposure to SWEEP, the Theta imbalance reduced to 4.6 %, the Alpha to 5.2 %, and the Theta/Beta ratio imbalance to 3.2 %.

A second example was a 14-year-old female with the Beta imbalance form of depression. Initially, her Beta amplitude imbalance in the frontal regions was 23.5 % with F4 being greater than F3. After a 10-min exposure to SWEEP, the imbalance reduced to 8.4 %. Again, the initial treatment with exposure to SWEEP was followed with neurofeedback uptraining of Beta at location F3.

A particularly effective treatment mix is to combine SWEEP with braindriving Theta or Alpha up at locations Pz or O1 or O2. This protocol has the effect of calming the person and improving subjective mood states. In contrast to the examples cited above, in the latter case, SWEEP is presented simultaneously with the Theta enhance braindriving.

Other forms of bilateral stimulation can be used in the same manner as SWEEP is used. The bilateral sound and vibration stimulators that EMDR therapists use can be used in the same manner as SWEEP. Tapping on the client's shoulders or knees, standard EMDR procedures, likewise can be used in place of the SWEEP harmonic for braindriving and the other applications described above.

The adjunctive treatment procedures described above are static in the sense that they are applied to have a specific effect on the autonomic and/or central nervous system functioning. The OMNI harmonic, for example, is prescribed for home use for a CADD child because at intake it has been determined that this stimulation will reduce Theta amplitude for this person.

Harmonics can be used both statically, such as listening to the sounds while doing homework, and contingently, such as hearing the sounds only under specific EEG conditions. The latter is a classical conditioning paradigm. When the brain wave amplitude rises above a specific threshold, for example, then a specific harmonic sound is presented that suppresses the amplitude of that brain wave. As will be described in detail later in this chapter, this procedure is remarkably effective when used with tasking behaviors that one is attempting to remediate. For example, if a poor reader has excessive Theta amplitude, then one can use the braindriving Theta suppress paradigm to suppress the Theta amplitude while the child is reading.

Chapter 6
Braindriving

Light and sound stimulation, which is used in Audiovisual Stimulation (AVS) devices, does affect brainwave activity. These devices are often preprogrammed to provide stimulation in the Theta or Alpha ranges to enhance quieting and relaxation. Stimulation in higher ranges or specifically in the high Alpha range is designed to improve cognitive functioning. AVS stimulation in the high Alpha range does result in localized increases in APF (Pfurtscheller et al. 1988), and stimulation close to one's own APF results in greater enhancement than stimulation rates that are double one's range (Frederick et al. 2005). It has also been shown that EEG changes associated with noncontingent (i.e., not contingent on EEG) AVS do not result in changes after the stimulation is terminated.

The protocols to be described in this section can be quite complex, in the sense that many contingencies can be associated with specific EEG events. One can have lights go on or off coincident with sounds going on or off or any other stimuli including electrical, electromagnetic, or vibration. The presentation or removal of these stimuli can likewise be complex. For example, the "push/grab" protocol could be the presentation of an Alpha-enhancing harmonic when the Alpha amplitude falls below some threshold, but an Alpha frequency light (e.g., 11 Hz) is presented when the Alpha amplitude is above threshold. The harmonic "pushes" the Alpha and the flashing light entrains the Alpha when the amplitude is above threshold.

For emergencies, when clients are in severe anxiety and distress, one generally uses slow frequency amplitude enablers. For example, one might have slow frequency lights presented when Beta amplitude exceeds threshold, a Theta-enhancing harmonic presented when Theta is below threshold, and electrical stimulation of acupuncture point P6 (Pericardium 6, on the dorsal surface of the wrist) when Theta amplitude is above threshold. The latter acupuncture stimulation point has been shown to enhance Theta amplitude in the occipital regions of the brain (Swingle 1998).

There are several products for delivering harmonics contingent on EEG or other biofeedback events. Many EEG feedback systems have built-in, or optional, methods for delivering light or sound stimulation contingent on the EEG. There are

P.G. Swingle, *Adding Neurotherapy to Your Practice*,
DOI 10.1007/978-3-319-15527-2_6

also several stand-alone products that will interface with any biofeedback system that has sound output. The stand-alone systems are simply sound-activated electronic gates that permit control of any on/off function of electrical devices. The devices can include light and sound systems, CD players, electrical stimulation sources, and even devices like electric trains and wireless toys.

There are also software products that will deliver specific sounds contingent on biofeedback events. Some of the major EEG platform manufacturers have braindriving options for delivering both sound and visual stimulation. Braindriving software suites are also offered by a variety of software companies that allow clinicians to program complex contingencies for light and sound stimulation.

The cases presented in this section were treated with protocols using the Braindryvr Cascade system. This is a stand-alone system that is an acoustic gate to present the stimulation contingent on EEG events. The acoustic gate is triggered by the sound output from the EEG (neurofeedback) system. The Braindryvr Cascade will work with any biofeedback system with sound output.

It would perhaps be useful at this point to offer a few examples of stimulating or braindriving the EEG. The most straightforward example is a child with CADD, in which the only remarkable feature of the ClinicalQ is high-amplitude Theta activity over the sensory motor cortex (location Cz). The usual treatment for this condition is Theta inhibit, Beta enhance neurofeedback over location Cz. The number of sessions required to treat this disorder using "conventional" neurofeedback is between 40 and 80 (Lubar 1991). One can reliably and permanently remediate this simplest form of ADD in 15–20 sessions using braindriving technology (Swingle 2001). In between one-third and one-half of the neurotherapy sessions, braindriving is included. When Theta amplitude is below the training threshold, the game icons move and the child hears the reward tone. When the Theta amplitude goes above the training threshold, then the game icons stop moving and the child does not hear the reward tone, but a Theta-suppressing harmonic is presented via the Braindryvr Cascade, which suppresses Theta amplitude.

A more complicated example is in the treatment of seizure disorders. A common treatment for epilepsy is to enhance the amplitude and/or frequency of SMR operant responses over the sensory motor cortex (locations C3, Cz, and C4). One should also set an inhibit on Theta because if Theta amplitude increases when the SMR amplitude increases, there is a likelihood that seizure activity will remain unchanged or become worse even though SMR amplitude is increasing (Lubar and Bahler 1976). Using braindriving technology, one can cascade the units so the Theta-suppressing harmonic is presented when Theta amplitude increases above threshold, and the SMR-enhancing harmonic is presented when SMR amplitude drops below threshold. The braindriving technology can be used alone (i.e., no visual feedback) or with visual feedback displays.

Prior to all braindriving sessions, the efficacy of the UCS should be assessed. Because braindriving is an aggressive therapy, the changes are often sizable, but one should expect some after session regression towards pretreatment levels. The resulting after treatment level is usually above pretreatment level. Often to stabilize the braindriving gains, the client is shifted to straightforward neurofeedback.

Braindriving can also be added to regular neurofeedback protocols by having the UCS sound as the feedback with the client instructed to keep the sound "off." If the UCS lights are presented on goggles with look-through lenses, the child can be reading, writing, doing math, etc. while the implicated area of the brain is under braindriving treatment. This has been found to be very effective for facilitating skill acquisition (e.g., written output).

In most cases, braindriving is not used exclusively in the treatment of any condition but is combined with conventional neurofeedback. This is a practical clinical decision since the method of researching this technology has been to add it to the neurotherapy, observe the changes in the EEG, and determine if the enhancements are sustained in the ongoing neurotherapy treatment sessions. There have been cases in which braindriving has been used exclusively but there have been cases in which there were circumstances mitigating conventional neurotherapy (e.g., severe autism).

Braindriving is particularly effective for treatment of infants. Prior to the use of classical conditioning protocols in neurotherapy, neurotherapists would not treat infants because they could not get adequate QEEG measurements, and more importantly, because they do not believe that neurofeedback could be effective because the child was not capable of volitional attention to the feedback contingencies. Braindriving can be used with any client whether or not they are capable of volitional attention and engagement in the process. Thus infants, demented adults, delayed children, and comatose patients can be treated with the braindriver methodologies.

The following two cases illustrate the use of braindriving with infants. The first was a 9-month-old male infant with West Syndrome, a condition characterized by infantile seizures. Prognosis is generally not good with these infants with some estimates of only about 5 % of treated children achieving relatively normal cognitive and motoric development. Treatment with vitamin B6 and the Ketogenic Diet has been found to be successful in addition to antiseizure medications. The latter, however, carries the potential for cognitive impairment or delay as a side effect.

This child came for intensive treatment (up to three sessions per day) for a 3-month period. Upon his arrival at the clinic, this child had no seizure-free days. His Theta/Beta ratios were 4.8 (Cz) and 5.9 (O1), and his Theta/SMR ratios exceeded 10 at all locations over the sensory motor cortex. Preliminary assessment of the Theta suppressive effect of OMNI indicated a 12.8 % decrease. Assessment of the EFT (the EFT procedure is described elsewhere in this book) acupuncture tapping treatment procedure indicated an increase in SMR of 55.7 % and an increase in Theta amplitude of 69.7 %. Assessment of EFT with OMNI indicated an increase of Theta amplitude of 16.0 % with SMR amplitude increase of 38 % indicating that home use of EFT with OMNI would efficaciously reduce the Theta/SMR amplitude ratio. The parents administered the EFT with OMNI protocol (three repetitions of the EFT sequence per session) at least 15 times per day during their stay in Vancouver. They were instructed to continue the home treatment at least five times per day after returning home following treatment at the clinic.

The braindriving protocol used for this infant was OMNI on when Theta amplitude was above threshold and vibration of a soft cuddly toy bear when the amplitude of SMR was above training threshold. One can debate whether the vibration of the soft toy was a reward (instrumental conditioning) or the application of an unconditioned stimulus (classical conditioning). The bear vibration did increase the amplitude of the SMR in pretest.

At the start of the treatment, the infant had no Seizure Free Days (SFD). After the first month of treatment, the child had 45.0 % SFD; at 2 months 57.1 % SFD; at 10 weeks 87.7 % SFD; at end of treatment after 3 months 100 % SFD.

The second case was a 22-month-old male child diagnosed with "genetic degenerative brain disorder" with infantile seizures and spasms. The child also had limited use of his arms. Although there are many degenerative brain disorders, the parents reported that their child's condition was terminal, and that the only therapeutic options were to, essentially, sedate and medicate to inhibit seizures until the child died. The parents wanted to try neurotherapy to control the seizures/spasms and to be able to minimize medications that had sedating effects so they could have a relationship with their child until he died. The parent's report of the child's condition was verified by the referring physician.

The treatment paradigm was similar to the above case of the infant with West Syndrome. At intake, the child's frontal Delta amplitude was 29.1; the Theta/SMR ratio was over 8 at all locations over the sensory motor cortex; summated 16–25 Hz and 28–40 Hz amplitudes at location Fz was 31.4. The treatment of this child included the home EFT protocol and Craniosacral Therapy (CST) as part of every in-office neurotherapy session. One such session, focused on decreasing the Theta/SMR amplitude ratio at location C4, included OMNI presented when Theta amplitude was above training threshold and vibration of the toy cuddly bear when SMR amplitude was above training threshold. At the start of the session, the Theta/SMR ratio was 6.20 and following the treatment session the ratio was 4.28, a change of −31 %. Follow-up report from the parents included: "child was alert and interactive; many seizure free days; regained partial use of arms; died 16 months after treatment."

Autism is a good example of conditions in which braindriving technology is particularly efficient. Many Autistic Spectrum Disorder (ASD) clients lack the capability to participate effectively in volitional forms of neurofeedback. They simply cannot attend to the feedback screens or feedback sounds. There is evidence, of course, that the simple sound feedback will result in learning with positive results. However, the braindriving techniques are markedly more efficient and effective because the client need not be attentive and the stimuli being contingently presented are classically conditioning the desired brainwave state. Hence, very severely disabled ASD clients can be effectively treated with braindriving techniques. As the ASD client progresses, the protocols are gradually shifted to more volitional paradigms. During the transitional phases, both braindriving and volitional neurofeedback paradigms are presented simultaneously.

Standard Braindriving Protocols

The protocols for braindriving can be exceedingly complex. One can program the braindrivers to present light, sound, electrical stimulation, vibration, and electromagnetic stimulation in a wide variety of combinations all of which are contingent on specific EEG events. In most clinical settings, the majority of clients can be efficiently treated with a few standard braindriving protocols.

The first decision that the clinician must make is whether to suppress or to increase brainwave amplitude. The second decision is to select the braindriving stimuli based on whether the stimuli are to suppress or to entrain the selected brainwave. For example, an 18 Hz flashing light can be used to suppress Theta if the onset of the light is made contingent on Theta amplitude exceeding some threshold. This same light frequency can, on the other hand, be used to enhance Beta amplitude if it is presented when Beta amplitude exceeds a training threshold. The former uses the 18 Hz light to suppress slow frequency amplitude, and the latter uses the 18 Hz to entrain Beta.

Several examples of braindriving protocols are shown in Figs. 6.1, 6.2, 6.3 and 6.4. Figure 6.1 shows the data associated with braindriving Beta down at location O1 for a client with a deficient Theta/Beta ratio. Common complaints associated with this condition, as previously discussed, include problems with stress tolerance, sleep quality, and self-medicating behavior. Concentration can also be poor because of "brain chatter." As the data indicate, contingent stimulation of the Heart 6 (palmer ulnar surface slightly above the wrist crease) acupuncture meridian (bilateral) resulted in a decrease in the amplitude of Beta and an increase in the amplitude of Theta. The resulting increase in the Theta/Beta ratio after this 20 min session was 76.1 %. Subjective reports following this session was of profound quiescence. Recall, the efficacy of the UCS for this client is pretested before the braindriving session.

Figure 6.2 shows the data from an elderly client who was experiencing problems with memory and cognitive efficiency. Alpha slowing, measured in this case with the Alpha density ratio of lo-Alpha/hi-Alpha, can be an age-related decline. These declines can be effectively treated with brain-brightening protocols such as those developed by the late Budzynski et al. (2007). Braindriving also has been shown to be particularly effective for these clients as the data shown in Fig. 6.2 indicate. The protocol was to present both the OMNI harmonic (a blend of sounds that reliably suppresses Theta amplitude) plus 11 Hz visual stimulation whenever 8–9 Hz brainwave amplitude crossed the training threshold. As indicated, the pretreatment L/H Alpha ratio was 2.83 which dropped to 2.76 after the first 2 min of treatment. By the end of treatment, the ratio was 1.78, which is a 37.1 % decrease. Further sessions, either neurofeedback or braindriving, would be required to bring this ratio into efficient range (below 1.50). Once the L/H Alpha ratio is in an acceptable range, clients with persistent age-related decline are assessed and treated between two and four times per year to maintain efficient Alpha peak frequency.

Fig. 6.1 Braindriving Beta down @ O1 with H6 stimulated>T

Pre-treatment Θ/β 0.85

	Θ	β	Θ/β
START	14.3	12.4	1.09
END	17.8	9.4	1.92
%	24.5	-24.2	76.1

Fig. 6.2 Braindriving low Alpha down @ Fz with OMNI and 11 Hz visual>T

Pre-treatment L/H α = 2.83

	Lα	Hα	L/Hα
START	14.1	5.0	2.76
END	10.0	5.6	1.78
%	-29.1	+12.0	-35.5

Fig. 6.3 Braindriving Theta down @ Cz with 16 Hz and OMNI>T

Pre-treatment Θ/β under cognitive challenge = 3.29

	Θ	β	Θ/β
START	23.5	7.4	3.17
END	18.8	8.4	2.23
%	-25.0	13.5	-29.6

Fig. 6.4 Braindriving Alpha @ Pz with 11 Hz and SERENE<T

Trauma Release

Trial	Θ	α	β	
1	12.5	11.5	8.2	
2	16.0	13.2	9.4	
3	13.1	15.5	9.9	← α release
4	8.4	12.6	9.3	emotional release
5	9.7	11.0	8.8	emotional release
6	9.2	10.9	8.6	emotional release
7	8.8	10.1	8.1	emotional release
8	12.9	12.9	9.1	recovery
9	15.8	13.4	9.5	recovery
10	14.7	15.2	9.5	recovery

Figure 6.3 shows a braindriving session with a client with the common ADD condition of elevated Theta amplitude as measured at location Cz. By the end of the session, the Theta/Beta ratio had decreased by about 30 %.

One very important use of braindriving is for treatment of emotional trauma. Obviously, this procedure should be used only by licensed providers experienced in dealing with clients affected by posttraumatic stress. The blunted Alpha response, discussed earlier, is a marker for unresolved emotional stress. There are several methods for releasing and processing this emotional state including EMDR, hypnosis, and experiential psychotherapies to mention but a few. Braindriving can markedly accelerate this process in a positively synergic manner.

The data shown in Fig. 6.4 show emotional release with one of the "Alpha push" protocols. As the data indicate, as the Alpha amplitude starts to increase, this client experienced an emotional release, lasting about 8 min. Many therapists stop the braindriving at this point and continue with a procedure such as EMDR or experiential therapy or simply letting the client silently experience the emotional release. In this case, the client continued with braindriving and started the recovery phase after about 8 min. After the session, the client was probed regarding the experience. She reported an emotional episode which she described in some detail. Brief therapeutic intervention resulted in an emotional redefinition of the event, a desired outcome of such therapy.

The following basic protocols are based on two available braindriving channels. If only one channel is available, the clinician can use one of the two features of each protocol depending on desired effects on brainwave amplitude.

For clinicians with two EEG systems and two braindrivers available, protocols can be used to drive two different areas of the brain simultaneously. For example, clients with depression who show one of the disparities in the frontal regions of the brain can have each of the two frontal lobes targeted independently. Sounds and lights can be presented to each ear and each eye independently to aggressively balance the brainwave amplitudes in the frontal cortex.

Although a more eloquent sounding terminology could be used, I have found in my clinic that the terms "Suppress," "Push," and "Grab" are never confused. Clinicians and technical staff all understand that "Suppress" means to reduce amplitude, "Push" means to enhance amplitude, and "Grab" means to catch elevated amplitude with an entraining stimulus to increase time above threshold.

Suppress/Suppress

In this preparation, both stimuli are designed to suppress brainwave amplitude. To suppress Theta, for example, one can have 18 Hz light stimulation presented through the LED goggles and an OMNI harmonic presented through headsets. As the name of this protocol implies, both the light and the sound stimuli are presented when Theta amplitude exceeds the training threshold. For an ADD child with excessive

Theta amplitude at location Cz, the stimuli would "go on" whenever the amplitude of Theta exceeded the training threshold. If the training threshold was set for 30 %, then the lights and the sound would come on during the 30 % of the time when Theta amplitude exceeded the specific threshold.

Push/Push

As the name implies, this procedure is designed to increase the amplitude of a specific brainwave. The set-up is exactly opposite to the suppress/suppress protocol. The stimuli designed to increase the amplitude of a specific brainwave would "go on" when the treatment brainwave is below the training threshold. For example, if the clinician wants to increase the amplitude of Alpha, then light stimulation, such as 11 Hz, and the SERENE harmonic would be presented whenever the amplitude of Alpha dropped below a threshold. In this case, the training threshold would be set around 70 % so that the lights and the harmonic are presented about 30 % of the time and the Alpha amplitude would be above threshold about 70 % of the time. As the percent time above threshold increases, the threshold value is increased to maintain the 70 % above threshold average.

Push/Grab

This is an effective procedure for increasing Theta amplitude for clients with traumatic stress, addictions, and anxiety disorders. The SERENE harmonic is presented whenever Theta amplitude drops below threshold, and a Theta frequency light (7.8 Hz appears to be especially effective) is presented whenever Theta amplitude is above threshold. The push/grab protocol can be used whenever the clinician has stimuli available that will entrain and augment a particular brainwave band. Combinations might include 11 Hz lights with SERENE for increasing Alpha amplitude, 18 Hz lights and OMNI to increase Beta amplitude, and 4 Hz lights and SERENE to increase Theta amplitude.

An example of the push/grab protocol is a 78-year-old male client who has a problem with excessive alcohol use and a sleep disturbance. At intake, this client's Theta/Beta ratio at location O1 was 0.54 and had increased to about 0.80 after some neurotherapy sessions. The ratio at O1 was 0.84 at the beginning of the braindriving session. The "push" stimulus was SERENE and the "grab" or entraining stimulus was 7.83 Hz lights. The lights were presented when Theta amplitude was above threshold, and SERENE was presented when Theta amplitude was below the training threshold. The session was 30 min in duration, and at the end, the client's ratio was 1.20, with an increase of 42.8 %.

Combinations with the SWEEP Harmonic

The SWEEP harmonic can be very effective when combined with any of the light frequencies. SWEEP balances the frontal brain regions, but it also has a soothing effect on many clients so it can be used for both attention- and focus-oriented treatments as well as relaxation-oriented treatment. Some common combinations include increasing Theta amplitude in the occipital regions with 7.8 Hz lights; increasing Alpha amplitude at Pz with 11 Hz lights; and decreasing HighBeta/Gamma at location Fz with 3 Hz lights.

Case Examples

Push Protocol As discussed above, the clinician may elect to use only a single stimulus for braindriving. In this case, for example, only one sound stimulus was used to "push" the Alpha amplitude. The client is a young woman under treatment for a severe anxiety disorder that manifested eating difficulties and poor immune functioning as evidenced by incessant colds and flus. Increasing Alpha amplitude in the occipital region of the brain (location Oz) has been shown to enhance immune functioning (increased CD4+ lymphocyte count) (Shummer et al. 2013).

Of several areas requiring treatment, one prominent brainwave feature was a markedly deficient Theta/Beta ratio at location O1. Her ratio was 0.57, whereas normative would be between 1.80 and 2.20. The neurotherapeutic treatment for this condition is to enhance Theta amplitude and/or decrease Beta amplitude at location O1. Generally, one does not commence treatment with these brainwave bands nor at that exact location but gradually approaches the training bandwidths and locations starting in areas and with bands that are easier for the client to master. Hence, training initially was to increase Alpha amplitude by braindriving the Alpha at location O1. The potentiating harmonic for Alpha amplitude enhancement, SERENE, was presented to the client anytime the Alpha amplitude dropped below the training threshold. The baseline Alpha amplitude was 3.2 microvolts (μV) which increased to 8.4 μV after 20 min of braindriving. Consistent with what one finds with Alpha/Theta neurofeedback training, when Alpha amplitude increases, Theta tends to increase as well. In this case, the Theta amplitude increased by 15.4 % (from 5.2 to 6.0 μV).

Push/Suppress The push/suppress protocol is used when one wants to suppress one brainwave range and enhance or "push" a second brainwave range. A good example of this situation is in the treatment of seizure disorders in which one wants to enhance the amplitude of the Sensory Motor Rhythm (SMR), which is 13–15 Hz, and suppress Theta amplitude.

The client in this case is a 50-year-old man who did not have a seizure disorder. He was under treatment for posttraumatic diffuse body pain and severe sleep quality difficulties, a condition that likely would be diagnosed as fibromyalgia in conventional medical/psychological practices. His initial ratio of Theta to SMR (13–15 Hz) was 4.40, whereas a normative range is below about 3.00. At the session to be reported here, his starting Theta/SMR ratio was 3.29. The braindriving protocol was to present the Theta-suppressing harmonic, OMNI, when Theta amplitude exceeded the training threshold and to present the SMR-enhancing harmonic, SERENE, when the amplitude of the SMR dropped below the training threshold. Baseline measurements at the start of the session indicated a Theta amplitude of 5.6 μV and SMR amplitude of 1.7 μV. At the end of the session, the Theta amplitude remained unchanged at 5.6 μV, but the amplitude of the SMR had increased to 4.0 μV for a ratio of 1.40. It is unusual to have large changes like this, but this case nicely shows that even with driving techniques, the brain "knows what it needs"—a concept most neurotherapists embrace, in that Theta remained unchanged while the SMR amplitude increased even though both were driven. This client reported a marked improvement in the diffuse body pain at the next session.

Suppress with Neurofeedback Braindriving can be combined with traditional neurofeedback to facilitate the training. In this case, the client was a little girl under treatment for a serious learning disorder. One of the things we noticed in her ClinicalQ was that the anterior cingulate gyrus was hyperactive. Her ratio of HiBeta (28–40 Hz) to Beta was 0.88 at intake, whereas normative was 0.45–0.55. Hyperactivity of this structure is related to obsessive/compulsive forms of behavior including stereotypy of thought, problems "letting go" of thoughts, stubbornness, and of particular concern in situations of learning disorders, often resistance to accepting different approaches to learning.

Braindriving with young children is often integrated into conventional biofeedback procedures because braindriving alone is rather boring. One simply sits there while the computer delivers sound (and/or other stimuli) about 30 % of the time. As described above, braindriving can be integrated into conventional biofeedback with visual computer displays. In this case, the neurofeedback display was Pacman, where an icon moves across the computer monitor eating up dots whenever the neurofeedback parameters are satisfied. Braindriving was added to this standard neurofeedback situation, in that when Pacman was not moving the braindriving sound stimulus was presented. This particular session with this little girl was rather late in treatment. Her HiBeta/Beta ratio was 0.59 at the start of this session. The suppressing harmonic was SERENE, and the feedback game display was Pacman. The braindriving harmonic was presented, on average, 30 % of the time. At the end of the treatment session, the client's HiBeta/Beta ratio had dropped to 0.53, which is well within normative range.

Suppress/Suppress One of the most exciting applications of braindriving is with clients who have limited capacity for volitional biofeedback. Although it is an axiom of neurotherapy that the brain learns even if the client is not paying attention, nonetheless neurofeedback is compromised when the client has such limited capacities. Such clients include the more severe autistic spectrum disordered, psychotic, and brain injured. We have used braindriving with such clients, many of whom have become capable of fully cooperative volitional neurofeedback. Braindriving protocols for such clients include: suppression of HiBeta and Beta amplitude over the anterior cingulate gyrus with autistic spectrum disordered children with a "hot midline"; so-called "squash" protocols that suppress the amplitude of all frequencies from 2 to 25 Hz for developmentally delayed and Fetal Alcohol Syndrome (FAS) children; and slow frequency suppress and "speed-up" Alpha protocols for stroke clients.

This child, who I will call Sammy, spent the first 45 min of his first appointment screaming and thrashing on my office floor, despite the heroic efforts of his parents. Fortunately, one of my staff members is a most talented young woman who works magic with these seemingly unapproachable children. She was able to habituate Sammy to tolerate electrodes on his head and to remain relatively quiet for a few minutes at a time, watching videos of animated cartoons. After Sammy became habituated to the electrodes to the extent of tolerating them for a few minutes at a time, we started the braindriving protocols and obtained a ClinicalQ. The braindriving protocols included suppression of HiBeta and Beta over the frontal midline (Fz), "squash" over the frontal (F3 and F4) and central (Cz) areas, and suppression of Theta amplitude over the occipital regions (O1 and O2) as well as centrally and frontally.

All of Sammy's preliminary braindriving protocols were Suppress. OMNI was used to suppress Theta at locations O1 and O2, F3 and F4, and Cz. OMNI was also the suppressing harmonic to reduce the amplitude across all the brainwave activity from 2 to 25 Hz at locations F3, F4, and Cz. Visual suppressing 11 Hz light stimulation was presented through the look-through glasses using the suppress protocol; that is, both the light and the sound were presented when the brainwave amplitude exceeded the training threshold.

During the braindriving sessions, Sammy was kept occupied by watching cartoons on a portable DVD player. Sammy's case nicely illustrates the value of braindriving techniques with a child who is not attentive to the neurofeedback screens but is kept focused on cartoons. Systems are available that make the cartoon images contingent on brainwave amplitude. For example, the cartoons would stop playing (would pause) if the Theta amplitude exceeded threshold and would resume when the Theta amplitude dropped below the training threshold. In our experience, this procedure is considerably less effective when compared with the braindriving procedure described in Sammy's case.

There have been some remarkable changes in Sammy. He converses in sentences, albeit awkward and clipped, interacts with peers, and, importantly, is capable of volitional neurofeedback where we are now addressing the anomalies found in his full 19 site QEEG. We started with the ClinicalQ after Sammy was able to tolerate a single electrode, and the ClinicalQ guided our braindriving protocols. Once Sammy was able to tolerate the full head cap, we proceeded to the full QEEG to guide his treatment.

Braindriving with Tasking

One of the most powerful applications of braindriving is in the context of tasking. Tasking simply means that we ask the child to read and summarize, or read and write a sentence or two about the paragraph that was just read, or do mathematical problems, or work on puzzles, or organize objects according to shape, or any other task that may be relevant to the child's academic inefficiencies.

Figure 6.5 shows the glasses that are worn by the child while doing tasking. There are lights around the periphery of the lens so that the lights can go on or off depending on brainwave amplitudes, as described above. The child can look right through the clear lenses, so the child can be reading or writing or doing math problems while the brain is being stimulated.

Figures 6.6 and 6.7 show the written output of a child who had been diagnosed as having a Written Output Disorder (WOD). Our thinking about WOD has changed much like our thinking about sleep disorders has changed. We now think of sleep problems as the cause, rather than as a symptom, of some other disorder, as we had in the past. For example, we now consider the sleep problem as the potential cause or exacerbater of depression rather than as a symptom of depression.

With WOD, it is the reverse. We now consider written output problems to be more of a symptom of some other disorder rather than a disorder in itself. Children have written output problems for a number of reasons, and the power of braindriving is that the area of the brain that is inefficient can be under direct treatment while the child is engaged in writing. So, we are treating the cause of the output problem and monitoring the symptom rather than trying to improve output by attempting to remediate the symptom with repetitive drills and the like.

As shown in Figs. 6.6 and 6.7, there was a marked change in this child's ability to write and communicate in written form. It is important to note that the change shown here took place over just three sessions.

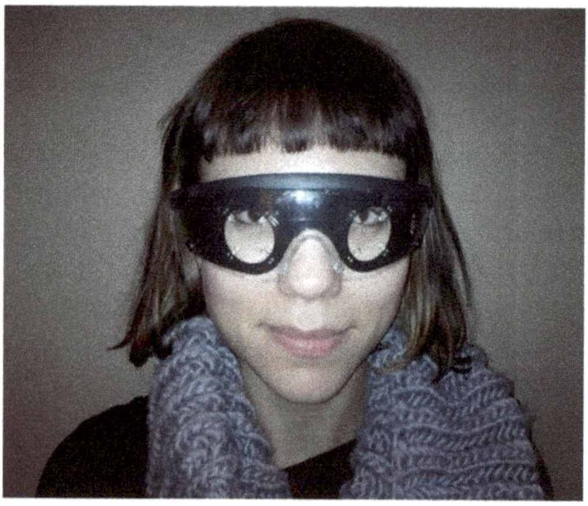

Fig. 6.5 Goggles for light stimulation used during braindriving tasking

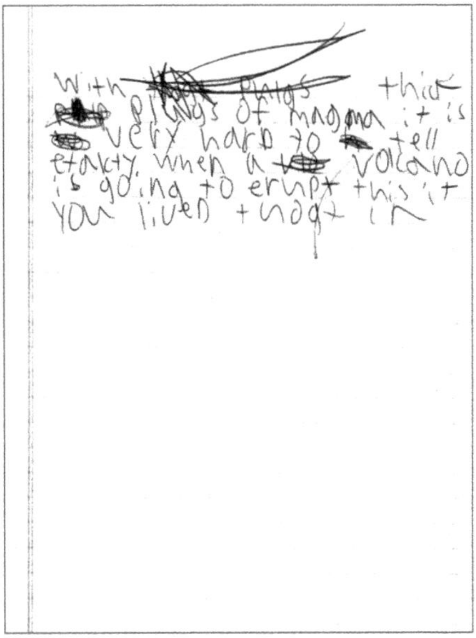

Fig. 6.6 First writing sample of child diagnosed with WOD

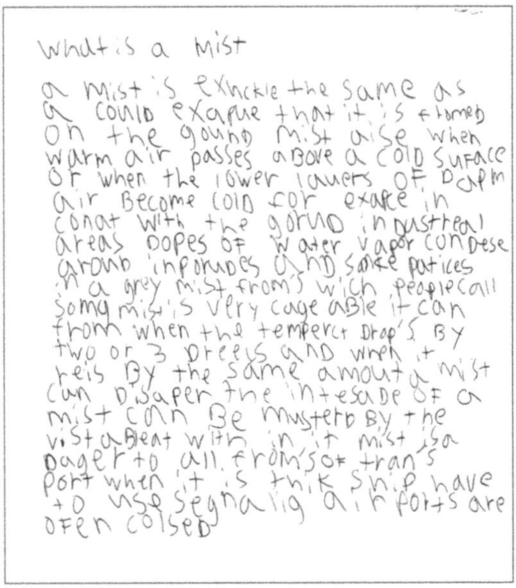

Fig. 6.7 Written output of child during third braindriving session

Emergency and Urgency Braindriving Protocols Emergency protocols are used to rapidly quiet severely distressed clients. In some cases, these clients are those under treatment who are experiencing decompensation, emotional abreactions, panic, or other severe emotional states. Others are new clients who come, or are brought, to you in states of emotional crises.

Table 6.1 Brief ClinicalQ procedure

Brief ClinicalQ
At location O1: Record Theta, Alpha, and Beta, both eyes open and eyes closed
At locations F3 and F4: Record Theta, Alpha, and Beta eyes closed
At location Fz: Record Delta, Lo-Alpha, Hi-Alpha, HiBeta-Gamma and Beta eyes closed
Delta (2 Hz)
Lo-Alpha (8–9 Hz)
Hi-Alpha (11–12 Hz)
Theta (3–7 Hz)
Alpha (8–12 Hz)
Beta (16–25 Hz)
HiBeta-Gamma (28–40 Hz)

In general, clients respond rapidly and well to these aggressive emergency protocols. However, if the client is heavily medicated, the effectiveness of these procedures can be markedly restricted. A case described later in this chapter shows the limited response of a heavily medicated client.

When dealing with a client presently under treatment, one knows the client's neurological condition, and the emergency protocol can be guided by the existing EEG data. For new clients, if possible, one should quickly assess the critical areas to determine the most efficient emergency protocol. The ClinicalQ can be reduced even further under such circumstances. The "brief" ClinicalQ is shown in Table 6.1.

Most clients in severe states of emotional distress will show a marked deficiency in the Theta/Beta ratio in the occipital region. The reason they are in distress is because of poor stress tolerance. If the ClinicalQ verifies this deficiency with a ratio well below 1.80, then the braindriving protocol should be focused on aggressively increasing Theta amplitude and/or decreasing Beta amplitude.

Push/Grab with SWEEP Urgency Protocol If the major feature of the ClinicalQ is the deficiency at O1, then the braindriving could be a "push–grab" protocol in which lights at 7.83 Hz are presented when the Theta is above threshold (grab), and the SERENE harmonic is presented when Theta is below threshold (push).

This protocol can also include electrical stimulation of acupuncture point P6 either continuously or when the Theta amplitude is below threshold (push). The electrical stimulation of acupuncture points is covered in the next section of this chapter.

If the ClinicalQ shows one of the depression markers in addition to the deficiency in the occiput, combining Theta enhance procedures with the SWEEP harmonic can be very effective. The depression markers are Theta or Alpha more than 15 % greater in the left relative to the right frontal cortex; Beta more than 15 % greater in the right relative to the left; or the Theta/Beta ratio more than 15 % higher in the left relative to the right cortex.

Theta amplitude can be enhanced in several ways. A particularly effective protocol for emergency conditions is to present the 7.8 Hz light stimulation when Theta is above threshold (grab). The SWEEP harmonic can also be presented continuously during the braindriving. The latter has the effect of balancing the frontal cortex. Thus, the procedure simultaneously quiets the client while balancing the frontal lobes to mitigate depressed mood state. As mentioned earlier, other methods of bilateral stimulation can be used in place of the SWEEP harmonic. The alternating tactile and/or alternating sound stimulation provided by the devices used by EMDR therapists work very effectively with this emergency protocol.

Several cases illustrate the use of this braindriving protocol for emergencies. All of these cases used 7.8 Hz light stimulation when Theta was above threshold (grab), mild electrical stimulation of P6 when Theta was below threshold (push), and continuous presentation of the SWEEP harmonic. In each of the cases presented, the client reported marked quieting and improved mood state after treatment. Their physical deportment and speech demeanor were consistent with their reports of relief from the distress.

Case A This client had been in treatment for 4 weeks and had completed three neurotherapy sessions. She requested emergency treatment because of uncontrollable crying and severe anxiety. Pretreatment brief ClinicalQ indicated a Theta/Beta ratio at location O1 of 1.30 and a disparity in the frontal lobes with the Theta/Beta ratio at F3 (2.38) being 41.7 % greater than the ratio at location F4 (1.68). The treatment protocol was braindriving to increase the Theta/Beta ratio at location O1 and to balance the frontal cortex. The electrode placement was at location O1; 7.8 Hz lights were presented when Theta was above the training threshold (grab), electrical stimulation of P6 was presented when Theta amplitude was below threshold (push), and SWEEP harmonic was presented continuously. The Theta/Beta ratio at location O1 increased by 66.9 % during treatment and the frontal lobe disparity reduced to 1.4 % after treatment.

Case B This 42-year-old male client was brought in by his sister because he was experiencing severe "unbearable anxiety." The client refused light stimulation because he claimed it caused a severe increase in stress. The protocol used in this case was electrical stimulation of acupuncture point P6 (see next section for a description of acustimulation procedures) when Theta was below training threshold (push) and presentation of the SERENE harmonic when Theta was below threshold (push). Pretreatment Theta/Beta ratio at location O1 was 0.96, and the posttreatment ratio was 1.94.

Case C One client, a 45-year-old female, reported severe depressed mood state with "frightening" suicidal thoughts. This client did not appear agitated and her Theta/Beta ratio at location O1 was consistent with this demeanor at 1.86. There was a disparity in the frontal lobes; the right (F4) had a Beta amplitude that was 15.8 % greater than the left (F3).

Two issues of particular interest in this case: First, note that the disparity in the frontal Beta amplitude is relatively minor, only 0.8 above the guideline. As stated earlier, the remarkable features in the ClinicalQ may not be large, but they are the salient markers for the client's seeking treatment. In this case, there were no other important anomalies in the brainwave data but the client presented with debilitating depression. The second point is that although frontal Beta is generally thought to be resistant to neurotherapeutic treatment, this emergency protocol demonstrates that such disparities are readily modified with braindriving procedures.

The protocol for this client was presentation of 18 Hz light stimulation when F3 Beta was below training threshold and presentation of the SWEEP harmonic on a continuous basis. Posttreatment disparity was 2.6 % (right greater than left), which is an 83.5 % change.

Contra Theta Urgency Protocol for Beta Suppression

Often clients arrive in states of severe angst or decompensation. When the Brief ClinicalQ indicates a severe excess of Beta amplitude at any of the critical sites (i.e., F3, F4, Fz, or O1), this excessive amplitude can often be aggressively suppressed by using Theta range stimulation. This is similar to the protocol using milligauss electromagnetic stimulation to reduce activation/arousal of an area (e.g., Fz) by contingently stimulating in Delta range when Beta amplitude exceeds the training threshold. This protocol using EMF stimulation was described earlier in this chapter.

The Contra protocol was developed based on evaluation of the low Theta amplitude correlations between locations F3 and F4 ($r=0.20$) in the frontal cortex; the negative correlations between Beta amplitude at locations F3 ($r=-0.28$) and F4 ($r=-0.31$) with Theta/Beta ratio at location O1 in the occipital region of the brain; the negative correlations between Beta amplitude at F3 ($r=-0.30$) and F4 ($r=-0.33$), and the Theta/Beta ratio at location Fz. Frontal Delta also correlates with frontal Theta (F3, $r=0.58$ and F4, $r=0.56$). All of the correlation coefficients are statistically reliable ($p<0.001$). (As discussed earlier in this book, it is interesting to note that the correlations among brain sites are different for the bipolar population of patients. To date, at the Swingle Clinic, the Contra protocols have not been used with the bipolar patients.)

Because of the negative correlations between the frontal regions (F3 and F4) and between these frontal sites and the two other critical areas commonly treated for Beta amplitude elevations (i.e., Fz and O1), visual stimulation at both ends of the Theta bandwidth range were presented independently to each eye. Contralateral sound was also initially used, but clinical evidence indicated that presenting the same sound frequencies to both ears simultaneously contingent on treatment threshold crossings was most efficacious. This protocol is effective for aggressive Beta amplitude reductions at locations Fz, F3, F4, and O1.

This complex braindriving protocol can be programmed on Mind Work Station, BioExplorer, and Braindryvr software suites. Using the Braindryvr Cascade or other computer add-on relay system with independent Audiovisual Stimulation units is also very effective.

The Contra Beta Suppress protocol is as follows: Below Beta amplitude training threshold: 7.8 Hz sound to both ears and 3 Hz visual stimulation to right eye. Above Beta amplitude training threshold: 3 Hz sound to both ears and 7.8 Hz visual stimulation to left eye.

The Contra Beta Suppress protocol is very aggressive and effective treatment for reducing Beta amplitude of the frontal and occipital regions. The following case

EPOCHS	THETA	BETA	ALPHA
1	11.8	9.9	7.4
2	10.0	8.6	6.9
5	8.2	7.8	6.9
9	10.6	7.4	6.8
10	11.3	7.7	6.9
PRE TX	10.6	18.3	8.3

Fig 6.8 Contra Beta suppress braindriving protocol at location F3

examples indicate the effectiveness of this procedure. It should be noted that because the Contra protocol is aggressively pushing Beta amplitude down, the amplitude will rise after treatment stops but usually remains well below pretreatment levels. Further, as indicated throughout this book, braindriving and other aggressive procedures are usually followed by later sessions of volitional neurofeedback to stabilize gains.

The following case shown in Fig. 6.8 is a 67-year-old female client reporting severe anxiety. Her ClinicalQ indicated, among other remarkable features, the frontal imbalance associated with poor stress tolerance and anxiety conditions. The Pretreatment (PRE TX) Beta imbalance between F3 and F4 was 49.5 % with the left being greater than the right. This case points out a number of issues associated with the aggressive Contra protocol. First, it is often observed that the major changes in brainwave amplitude occur within the initial few minutes of treatment. The epochs in this treatment protocol were 2 min each indicating that the change from PRE TX level of Beta amplitude was 45.9 % after the first 2 min of treatment. The remaining 18 min of treatment resulted in an additional amplitude reduction of 22.2 %. Also, as indicated in the figure, the major Beta suppression had been achieved by epoch 5.

Elevated Beta and High Beta-Gamma amplitude at location Fz also respond very favorably to the Contra Beta suppress protocol. As discussed in the previous chapter, elevated fast frequency amplitude in this area of the brain is associated with client reports of perseverative though processes, fretting, and anxiety. Elevated activity in this region is also often found to exacerbate other conditions such as depression.

The following case (Fig. 6.9) is a 31-year-old male who was reported to have severe anxiety, anger outbursts, and psychotic states. His pretreatment HighBeta-Gamma (28–40 Hz)/Beta (16–25 Hz) (HBG/B) ratio was 0.93, and the summation of the two amplitudes was 16.2 μV.

The training range was 13–40 Hz with the same contingencies as described above (7.8 Hz sound to both ears and 3 Hz visual stimulation to right eye. Above training Beta range (13–40 Hz) amplitude training threshold: 3 Hz sound to both ears and 7.8 Hz visual stimulation to left eye).

As the data indicate there were very substantial reductions in both Beta ranges over the 20 min training session. Reduction of Beta amplitude in this region of the brain is often difficult and can require many sessions. The pretreatment HBG/B ratio

Fig. 6.9 Contra Beta suppress braindriving protocol at location Fz

EPOCHS	28-40Hz	13-40Hz	16-28Hz
1	7.1	12.0	7.8
2	5.7	10.5	7.1
5	5.4	9.9	6.7
9	4.5	9.4	6.5
10	4.9	9.8	6.7
PRE TX	7.8	12.2	8.4

was 0.93 which dropped to 0.80 after 10 min of treatment and was 0.73 at the end of the treatment session. This is still somewhat elevated and the goal in future sessions was to bring this ratio down to below 0.60. The amplitude summation was 16.2 prior to treatment, 12.1 at epoch 5, and 11.6 at the end of the treatment session.

Contra Protocol to Increase Alpha Peak Frequency

As discussed in the section on synergy between medicine and neurotherapy, Alpha Peak Frequency (APF) is an indicator of brain efficiency. It appears as though increasing fast Alpha and decreasing slow Alpha have beneficial effects on all aspects of cognitive functioning. Better performance is associated with elevated fast Alpha, even for clients with Alzheimer's (Klimesch 1999). As well, efficacy of many medications is associated with faster APF. Many of the braindriving protocols for increasing APF use suppress low Alpha amplitude (8–9 Hz) and/or push high Alpha amplitude (11–12 Hz). The principle reason is for braindriving efficiency, although there is evidence to suggest that training down low frequency Alpha amplitude may have benefit in addition to increasing mean Alpha frequency (Zoefel et al. 2011).

The protocol is as follows: Train High Alpha (11–12 Hz). Below Threshold, 11 Hz sound to both ears, 10 Hz visual stimulation to the right eye. Above Threshold, 10 Hz sound to both ears, 11 Hz visual stimulation to the left eye.

As shown in Fig. 6.10, the Low/High Alpha ratio was 3.03 at pretreatment baseline and was reduced to 1.43 after the 20 min braindriving treatment. This is a reduction of 52.8 %. As described above, the density ratio of low to high Alpha is used to facilitate the braindriving protocol. Follow-up stabilization sessions are generally regular neurofeedback rewarding increases in Alpha Peak Frequency. Recall, the correlation between the Low/High Alpha ratio and APF is $r=0.81$.

A study of veterans with PTSD found elevated APF which suggests that APF may be associated with hypervigilance (Wahbeh and Oken 2013). Also, the no-PTSD group had similar APF on both frontal areas, while the PTSD group had a higher

Fig. 6.10 Contra low Alpha suppress braindriving protocol at location Fz

EPOCHS	High Alpha	Low Alpha	Alpha
1	3.6	10.1	11.8
2	3.4	12.0	13.6
5	3.1	9.0	8.8
9	3.4	4.8	6.9
10	3.5	5.0	6.8
PRE TX	3.6	10.9	13.3

APF on the right than the left. Hence, this APF braindriving procedure should be used with additional caution with the PTSD patients and may not be appropriate for some clients with history of exposure to severe emotional stress.

Braindriving Other Modalities

As discussed in an earlier section of this book, many stimuli have reliable effects on brainwave activity. Braindriving can be done with a wide variety of different stimuli that can enhance or suppress brainwave amplitudes. In addition, these techniques can be used to drive other physiological systems as well. In the following section, the use of braindriving technology with electro-acupuncture and with blood flow hemoencephalography (HEG) (Tinius 2004) will be discussed.

Push with Electro-Acupuncture During my training in acupuncture at an institute affiliated with the major psychiatric hospital in Shanghai, I was taught a number of acupuncture sites that were used for "mental problems." Some of these sites were defined as "heuristic," in the sense that they were used because they worked, not because they fit with acupuncture theory. Some of the sites were conventional, frequently used locations, such as Pericardium 6 (P6), Spleen 6 (SP6), and Du (Governor Vessel) 26.

Pericardium 6 is a particularly useful acupuncture site in the treatment of anxiety-based disorders. This site is located three finger widths up from the crease in the wrist in the center of the dorsal forearm. The site is under the tip of the third finger when placed on the forearm starting at the wrist crease. This bilateral site (same location on both arms) is the site that is stimulated by the wristbands that are used for motion sickness. Mild electrical stimulation (less than 1 mA) in the 20 Hz frequency range has the effect of increasing Theta amplitude as measured at the occipital sites (O1 and O2). Typical increases in amplitude are in the 5–10 % range (Swingle 1995, February).

Although the original work was done at 20 Hz, other electrical frequencies have been found to be effective as well. For example, a double pulsing protocol of brief bursts at 2 Hz followed by 12 Hz was used for a client experiencing a severe episode of Obsessive Compulsive Disorder (OCD) behaviors. As with many OCD clients, this young woman had a deficiency of Theta amplitude relative to Beta amplitude in the occipital region of the brain. At the time of this treatment, her Theta/Beta ratio was 1.07. After a 15-min treatment at P6 with the above electrical protocol, her Theta/Beta ratio increased to 1.60, for an increase of 49.5 %. Note that no other neurotherapy treatment was used in this case other than the electrical stimulation of the acupuncture point P6, bilaterally. Because of the effect of stimulation of this point on Theta amplitude in the back of the brain, it is often included as an adjunct to Alpha/Theta training at O1 or O2 to augment treatment. Such was the case with this client in that after the 15-min pretreatment, Alpha/Theta training was done for an additional 20 min to stabilize the gain in Theta amplitude.

Braindriving with Electromagnetic Stimulation

The amplitude of the Electromagnetic Field (EMF) used in braindriving is a fraction of the very powerful electromagnets used for the treatment of depression. Typically, for braindriving, the strength of the EMF is below about 400 mg or less than about 0.00006 of the commercial units used for treatment of depression.

There are a number of neurotherapy devices/systems that make use of these micro-strength levels of stimulation. The important feature of these systems, including braindriving, is contingency. Rather than the stimulation being chronic, lasting for several minutes, the stimulation is strictly contingent on some brain activity. At such low level, it is likely that the EMF stimulation does not influence action potentials but rather is a source of feedback information for the brain. It may also induce some entraining effect based on pulse frequency of the EMF field. For example, if the EMF is pulsating at 2 Hz whenever Delta (1–3 Hz) amplitude drops below training threshold, the amplitude may be enhanced because of entrainment. This in turn may reduce the activity level of the cortical structure under treatment. A good example of this is when the activity of the client's anterior cingulate gyrus is elevated. Instead of down training 28–40 Hz, one might have better success by increasing Delta amplitude at that same location.

For braindriving, the stimulation frequency of the EMF can be programmed from very slow (e.g., 0.1 Hz) to very fast (e.g., 100) depending on the duty cycle of the electromagnetic coils (i.e., how fast they can turn on and off). In practice, using braindriving protocols, the frequencies rarely go below 0.5 Hz or above 50 Hz.

One application of the EMF stimulation in braindriving is when clients have negative reactions to visual stimulation or have vulnerability to seizures. In one case, a client reported having a severe headache for 5 days that did not lessen with reasonable levels of a pain medication. She was under treatment for anxiety-related symptoms including major problems with sleep. A sleep assessment indicated deficient deep sleep, where her 4-day average sleep was only about 13 min per night. The eyes closed Theta/Beta ratio at the O1 site was 0.98, which would be consistent with the deficient deep sleep. This client was also very sensitive to visual stimulation, particularly with the headache, so magnetic stimulation was used to reduce the Beta amplitude using the suppress braindriving protocol. One Beta suppress protocol that has been found to be particularly effective is visual stimulation at 3 Hz when Beta is below training threshold and 7.8 Hz when Beta amplitude is above training threshold. In the present case, the magnetic stimulation frequencies were set as described above when used with visual stimulation. After a 15 min session, the Theta amplitude stayed about the same (Pre: 10.3 μV, Post: 10.8 μV). Beta amplitude dropped 20.7 % (Pre: 10.5 μV, Post: 8.7 μV). This resulted in an increase in the Theta/Beta ratio of 26.5 %. Other interventions were used in this case as well to reduce autonomic arousal.

Braindriving with Hemoencephalography

Braindriving with Hemoence-phalography (HEG) is a measure of local blood flow in the brain. It is based on the differences in tissue absorption of red and infrared light dependent on the concentration of oxygenated hemoglobin. Developed by Dr. Hershel Toomim (Toomim et al. 2004), this property of measured blood flow is the basis for HEG, that is, blood flow biofeedback of targeted areas of the brain. This increased oxygenation of brain tissues results in improvements in attention, recovery of function, reduced migraine headache, and improvements in attention.

In the treatment of ASD, severe developmental delays, severe FAS, and the like, HEG can be a useful treatment to activate the frontal regions of the brain. As with conventional neurofeedback, some severely disabled clients may not be capable of attending to the feedback for HEG. We found that using the OMNI harmonic with the braindriving technology can drive HEG as well.

HEG can be driven with light stimulation at 18 Hz and sound stimulation with the OMNI harmonic using the "Push/Push" protocol. In this protocol, the stimuli are presented whenever the HEG drops below training threshold. In a group of adult and child clients with severe ASD conditions, the average increase in the HEG was 4.9 % with a standard deviation of 3.9 for brief braindriving epochs of 2–5 min in length with the sensors placed over site Fp1.

The above cases give examples of the use of braindriving in different clinical situations. This section ends with a few other examples of braindriving under different conditions. With braindriving, we often find that the major effect occurs within the first few minutes and that prolonged treatment (20–30 min) yields minimal further gain.

The following data are from a session with a severely traumatized woman in which the purpose of the session was to increase Theta amplitude in the back of the brain (location O1). Her Theta amplitude was 3.6 μV when she started. The data for the first 20 s of treatment indicate that the Theta amplitude increased at 5 s intervals as follows: 4.1, 4.6, 5.8, and 8.1. Thus, after 20 s of braindriving her, Theta amplitude increased from 3.6 to 8.1 μV. After an additional 20 min, her Theta amplitude increased to 10.1 μV, indicating that the amplitude had increased 125 % in 20 s and an additional 24.7 % after an additional 20 min.

The client, a man in his 40s, was under treatment for anxiety, depression, and sleep disturbance. As is often the case, initial focus was on improving quality of sleep. Theta amplitude in the back of the brain (O1) was braindriven to increase the Theta/Beta ratio to reduce the sleep problem.

The protocol used was "Push/Grab" in which SERENE was presented whenever Theta dropped below threshold, and 7.83 Hz light was presented whenever Theta was above threshold. The end session data indicated that Alpha had decreased by 22.4 %, Beta by 17.5 %, but Theta had increased by 10.5 %. The Theta/Beta ratio at the start of the session was 1.00 and had increased to 1.34 by session end.

The final example is from a session in which the client, a woman in her 50s, had a braindriving session when she was heavily medicated with paroxetine (Paxil) and risperidone (Risperdal). At the start of the session, her Theta, Alpha, and Beta amplitudes were 3.1, 2.9, and 8.2, respectively. At the end of the 30 min session, the amplitudes were 3.0, 2.9, and 8.3, respectively. Thus, braindriving appeared to be ineffective under this condition, a situation often encountered, in my experience, with conventional neurofeedback with heavily medicated clients.

Braindriving Supportive of Other Therapies

The final case is a man who was physically beaten and later developed what was diagnosed as fibromyalgia. The data on treatment of fibromyalgia seem quite clear. Medications are not identified by patients as very helpful (other than treating comorbid depression) but are identified by patients as source of side effects whereas, exercise and cognitive therapies are rated as most effective treatments of all (Nüesch et al. 2013).

Glenn was a 67-year-old male who was physically attacked and beaten about the head, shoulders, and neck. Pain started in head, neck, and shoulders and then moved to other body locations. Major complaints: sleep disturbance, poor concentration, memory loss, inability to organize tasks and to concentrate, depression, fatigue, irritable, loss of libido, and right hand neuropathy.

Often neurotherapy is adjunctive to other treatments as a method for increasing the efficiency of those treatments. The treatment of fibromyalgia is generally a longer term therapy and one in which neurotherapy potentiates other treatment methods. In Glenn's case, the major therapeutic goal was to improve his sleep, as is generally the case with all fibromyalgia patients.

Second, exercise and muscles exercises have been found to be more effective than medications for helping clients with this condition, so Glenn was given several home treatment procedures for this purpose. For the sleep, Glenn was prescribed a Cranial Electrical Stimulator (CES), which has been approved for treatment of sleep (also depression and anxiety), which he was to use daily for at least 20 min.

He was also provided a pedometer to record the number of steps he walked every day. His preliminary activity was about 4,200 steps per day at the outset of treatment. He understood that an inactive person walks less than 5,000 steps per day and that the target for an active person is over 10,000 steps per day.

Finally, Glenn was also given a recording for guided Progressive Muscle Relaxation (PMR) and a second exercise version (cognitive tension reduction),

Table 6.2 Treatment of posttraumatic fibromyalgia

Home treatment				
CES				
PMR/CTR (Soothe)				
Pedometer				
Neurotherapy treatment				
Braindriving				
SMR up @ Cz; low Alpha down @ Fz				
Sleep log		Visits	Pain	No pain
Month	Hours	(1 h)	(Locations × occasions)	(days)
Jan	5.12	0	112	0
Feb	5.68	0	126	0
Mar	5.85	3	86	5
Apr	5.95	1	40	17
May	6.02	2	36	18
Jun	5.99	1	53	14
Jul	6.09	0	21	22
Aug	6.09	0	28	21
Sep	6.09	1	94	15
Oct	6.01	0	46	21
Nov	6.37	1	27	21
Dec	6.23	0	31	23

which essentially is guided mental imaging of tightening and releasing the same muscle groups as in the PMR exercise.

Table 6.2 shows the results of Glenn's record of sleep and pain. Treatment started in March and continued for about 9 months. As the data indicate, Glenn's sleep improved by about 1 h per night and he went from no pain free days to over 70 % pain free days. Glenn continued with the home treatments but only came for neurotherapeutic check-ups about every 9 months. These check-ups are more for monitoring any age-related declines in cognitive efficiency than for his fibromyalgia.

In summary, braindriving has been found to be an effective method for increasing the efficiency of neurotherapy. Combined with the very rapid and efficient ClinicalQ intake procedure, neurotherapy can be a cost effective treatment option for a very wide range of disorders. Braindriving is simply applied learning theory in which stimuli with known and measurable effects on the central nervous system are made contingent upon a response, following a classical conditioning paradigm. This classical conditioning protocol can be combined with the operant conditioning properties of neurofeedback. In my opinion, the combination of volitional and non-volitional procedures described in this book will lead to the development of neurotherapy protocols that will be primary treatment options for many disorders.

Finally, quieting braindriving protocols can be extremely soporific so the therapist should be attentive to brainwave activity indicating that the client is falling

Average Amplitudes:	**THETA**	**ALPHA**	**BETA**
Trial #	Filter 1 uV	Filter 2 uV	Filter 3 uV
1	14.6	18.1	11.2
2	10.4	18.0	12.1
3	7.3	22.8	12.0
4	9.1	18.8	11.1
5	7.4	17.2	10.5
6	8.5	10.2	7.7
7	9.6	6.9	6.8
8	11.2	8.2	7.6
9	12.7	8.2	7.8
10	14.7	9.7	9.3
Session Avg.	10.5	13.8	9.6

Fig. 6.11 EEG of client going into sleep state

asleep. Figure 6.11 shows just such a client where Alpha and Beta drop substantially, while Theta starts to increase. The remarkable increase in the occipital Theta/Beta ratio in this case is attributable to the client's sleep state even though braindriving induced it.

Although it may be very tempting to interpret these data as indicating that the braindriving had markedly improved the client's Theta/Beta problem in the occipital region of the brain, alas, it is largely the change one would expect in sleep. If one calculates the increase in the Theta/Beta ratio from the first to the last epoch, the change is 21.5 %. If one calculates the change from the second epoch to the next to last epoch (often therapists will use these epochs to avoid start/stop artifact in data), the apparent improvement is a whopping 91.8 %!

Obviously to determine the actual benefit of the braindriving, if any, one would need to assess the Theta/Beta ratio after the client recovers from the sleep state. In this case, the reassessment of this ratio about 5 min after she awakened indicated a positive change of 11.2 %. Reassessment of this same ratio at the beginning of her next treatment session, 8 days later, indicated that the improvement was 9.8 %.

One of the risk factors associated with inducing profound relaxation/sleep in clients is what I call the "Spa Effect." I am emphatic with clients that coming to the clinic for treatment is not to make them feel good in a manner similar to what they would expect in at a spa or from having alcohol or a drug. The purpose is to change their neurological state to correct the condition causing the problem(s) for which they sought treatment. They should not evaluate treatment efficacy based on how they feel immediately posttreatment. Making them feel good is not the treatment goal; correcting the putative mechanism associated with their condition is the treatment goal.

This risk of Spa Effect is particularly problematic when very severely distraught clients are calmed with one of the aggressive braindriving quieting protocols. Clients can fixate on "I want to feel the way I did after that XXX treatment."

Of course, there is nothing negative about relaxation, but one must also attend to the grunt work of changing brain functioning. Clinically, one often compromises with splitting sessions so that the grunt work comes first and the reward comes after. Again, as stated repeatedly in this book; don't take off your clinical hat when embarking on neurotherapy. The "soft" therapy may well be the most important part of the treatment mix.

Chapter 7
Peripheral Biofeedback

Earlier in this book, I made reference to the biofeedback of other autonomic nervous system modalities including muscle tension, thermal (peripheral blood flow), electrodermal activity, and heart rate variability (HRV). These peripheral biofeedback treatments are often used prior to doing neurotherapy for the purpose of quieting and relaxing the client.

There are some conditions in which the treatment of choice is not neurotherapy but rather biofeedback of a peripheral modality. Tension headache is a good example of a condition that may respond more rapidly and efficiently to muscle (electromyographic) biofeedback than to brain wave biofeedback. Likewise, the treatment of migraine headache may respond more efficiently to peripheral blood flow training.

There are also some conditions that respond most favorably to a combination of both central and peripheral biofeedback, both sequentially and simultaneously. For example, HRV training has been shown to increase the amplitude of the sensory motor rhythm (13–15 Hz; SMR) (Reid and Nihon 2011; Reid et al. 2013). Thompson and Thompson (2011) report that simultaneous neurofeedback training to increase SMR amplitude over the sensory motor cortex (location Cz) combined with HRV training was very effective for the treatment of a client with advanced Parkinson's disease. Other peripheral biofeedback modalities were also used with this client to facilitate relaxation and concentration.

In the following paragraphs, I introduce some of these modalities for the practitioner. The following is limited to a basic introduction and description of biofeedback procedures of the autonomic system. It does not provide details adequate for a practitioner to learn these techniques. The interested clinician should read the definitive text in the area of biofeedback for the autonomic system by Schwartz and Andrasik (2005). Biofeedback texts, training manuals, and tutorial videos are available on the Association for Applied Psychophysiology and Biofeedback web store at www.aapb.org.

P.G. Swingle, *Adding Neurotherapy to Your Practice*,
DOI 10.1007/978-3-319-15527-2_7

Electromyographic (EMG) biofeedback provides information on the tension of the muscles. The tension level of a particular muscle group, as measured by the electrical activity, can be fed back directly to the client. The direct feedback helps the client learn how to relax the muscle tension. EMG biofeedback is valuable in the treatment of motor disorders with clients who have traumatic brain injury, such as a stroke. It also eases muscle pain problems, including lower back pain and headaches. Neurotherapists also frequently use EMG feedback of the muscles of the forehead as a general relaxation treatment.

Gruber and Taub (1998) showed that animal subjects could control various physiological systems. In one study they report that adult male monkeys could reduce muscle tension in the forearm of the dominant arm by an average of 50 % over a ten-session training period.

The following is the case of a client who was more effectively treated with peripheral biofeedback rather than with neurotherapy. The client, a male in his 40s, had been hospitalized because he was suicidal and depressed. For the past 5 years, he had suffered from a condition that started as a persistent headache and subsequently was experienced as a feeling of pressure and profound cognitive "fuzziness." He was in continuous discomfort, could not think properly, and had lost his job. He became increasingly withdrawn from friends and family and experienced frequent and intense episodes of depression with strong suicidal fantasies.

Numerous diagnostic tests had failed to identify the cause of his problem, so he was referred to me to determine if neurotherapy might help. The various brain scan procedures that he had received did not show anything extraordinary, so I decided to do some measurements of the peripheral system because the symptoms suggested that the peripheral autonomic nervous system, rather than the central nervous system, should be examined. The peripheral systems included the muscles, vascular system, heart functions, skin response, and breathing. The client's muscle tension, peripheral blood flow (as measured by skin surface temperature), electrodermal response, heart rate, and breathing were measured both at rest and when he was exposed to a minor stressor. The stressor that I generally use is backward serial sevens in which the client counts backward by sevens from some arbitrary number such as 713. The counting is done out loud. This procedure increases the heart rate, blood pressure, and other indicators of peripheral arousal.

The assessment provides a lot of information about the client's autonomic nervous system's level of arousal. At rest, the forehead muscle tension was 7.8 μV, and it increased to 12.8 μV when counting backward. The tension in the forehead should be around 2 μV and, when the client is counting, the increase should be in the range of 1.5 μV. The client's other autonomic systems indicated normal levels and normal reactions to stress.

It seemed likely that the problem was caused by excessive tension in the muscles of the head. To test this assumption, I had the client do muscle biofeedback of the muscles in the head and also in the muscles of his upper torso. The client was able to substantially reduce the muscle tension in his forehead in a short time. As the muscle tension decreased, skin conductance increased remarkably. Electrodermal activity responds to emotional feelings and in this case it occurred when he started to cry. I asked him about his crying, and he told me, "The pressure in my head is gone."

This client's problem was essentially a tension headache. Because he experienced this discomfort as pressure and "fuzziness" in the head rather than head pain, the tension headache was not diagnosed. Further, since his depression was a reaction to the discomfort in his head and not neurologically based, antidepressant medication was largely ineffective.

This client's treatment consisted of a few sessions of muscle biofeedback to teach him how to recognize when his muscles were tense and how to relax them. I also taught him some muscle relaxation exercises for home use. In addition, he needed psychological therapy and counseling to help him plan his reentry into social and work environments.

Treating the problem directly with muscle relaxation was clearly the most effective treatment. It should be noted that this client's response to the muscle tension biofeedback was very unusual. It is extraordinarily unusual for a client to respond so rapidly. Normally it would require many sessions for a client to reduce the tension to a level at which a beneficial change in the symptom would be reported.

Peripheral blood flow is the blood volume in the arterioles and venules near the skin surface. Blood flow can be measured in several ways, including by the blood pulse volume or, more generally, by the surface body temperature. As blood flow increases, surface body temperature increases. Blood flow and temperature biofeedback are effective treatment methods for enhancing body relaxation.

In the study described earlier, Taub has shown that monkeys can change their hand temperature with thermal biofeedback. The monkeys were first trained to increase their hand temperature. After 25 sessions the average change in hand temperature was 1.8° (F). The monkeys were then taught to lower the hand temperature. After 25 sessions the hand temperature dropped by not only the 1.8° increase but by an additional 0.7° (F) below the animals' original starting temperature. In clinical practice, it is more difficult for clients to lower their hand temperature than to raise it.

Setting up hand-warming biofeedback is simple. Basically, information about hand temperature is fed back to the client. The skin surface transducers are very sensitive, so temperature changes are rapidly fed back to the client. Clients can see the immediate results of their efforts to change their hand temperature. Through trial and error, patients soon learn how to focus their attention on their hands and experience a gradual sensation of warmth. Feelings of calm normally accompany the increasing hand warmth.

Hand-warming is often used as the first step in many neurotherapy treatments. For example, clients with severe anxiety are treated with brain wave biofeedback to increase the amplitude of Theta brain waves in the back of the brain. This treatment can often be speeded up if the client is first trained to increase hand temperature, which has a relaxing effect. This is often used prior to neurotherapy in the treatment of some forms of alcoholism as well. The client is first taught to increase hand temperature to calm the autonomic nervous system. After several successful sessions, neurofeedback of slow-wave activity in the back of the brain begins.

Thermal biofeedback is also effective in treating vascular disorders such as migraine headache, Raynaud's disease, and hypertension. It can also be used to treat some sleep disorders, such as nocturnal myoclonus (restless legs syndrome), which are related to reduced blood flow in the legs and feet.

Electrodermal biofeedback is another useful treatment. When one becomes aroused (e.g., thinking about something exciting, being startled by a loud noise, etc.), the electrical resistance of the skin drops as sweat glands are activated. The skin is a remarkably responsive organ and reflects subtle changes in emotions and sympathetic and parasympathetic stimulation, such as abrupt changes in breathing. Frequently used to help relaxation, the electrodermal response (EDR) can be a remarkably sensitive indicator of the emotional significance of thoughts, ideas, and memories. In psychotherapy sessions, the EDR is used to indicate the emotional significance of the issues being discussed. Often, the full emotional significance of a conscious thought is not obvious to the client. The EDR in such cases can reveal latent emotional dispositions that need to be discussed during therapy.

Heart rate variability (HRV) biofeedback teaches clients to identify the breathing frequency (resonance frequency, RF) to maximize respiratory sinus arrhythmia (RSA). Heart rate increases at inhalation and decreases during exhalation and is maximized at specific RF. The baroreflexes associated with the baroreceptors in the blood vessels in the neck, the carotid artery and the aorta, control blood pressure. When heart rate increases, blood pressure decreases and vice versa. HRV biofeedback increasing the RSA has stimulating effects on the vagus nerve, thus decreasing blood vessel inflammation. Such inflammation has been identified as a contributing factor to cardiovascular disorders (Kalogeropoulos et al. 2012). HRV biofeedback has been shown to be effective in the treatment of high blood pressure, asthma, emphysema, anxiety, and depression (Lehrer 2013).

The HRV treatment modality is often used in conjunction with neurotherapy. Reid et al. (2013), for example, assessed EEG changes in 40 clinical subjects, who were being treated with HRV in addition to neurofeedback. Clients showing successful HRV training (peak frequency heart rate between 0.05 and 0.15 Hz) also showed significant increases in SMR amplitude at location Cz. Conversely, Bazanova et al. (2013) trained high Alpha EEG (10–12 Hz) to measure its effect on HRV. They found that healthy male subjects with low resting levels of Alpha who increased Alpha had lowered EMG and greater HRV and showed increases in cognitive performance. Prinloo et al. (2013) examined the EEG correlates of HRV intervention in subjects exposed to experimental laboratory stress. After a single session of HRV BFB, significant changes were found with reduced Beta and increased Theta at the three central sites Fz, Cz, and Pz. The authors suggest these EEG changes indicate increased relaxation and decreased anxiety.

Biofeedback treatment can address many other medical issues. These biofeedback modalities include heart rate, heart rhythm, blood pressure, blood pulse volume, respiration rate, pupil dilation, and voice characteristics. All of these can be used in conjunction with neurotherapy.

Appendices

The following appendices contain summaries, forms, and information brochures that readers may duplicate and use in their practices:

Appendix A: Summary of the ClinicalQ
Appendix B: Bloodless Brain Surgery
Appendix C: Child Intake Questionnaire
Appendix D: Adult Intake Questionnaire
Appendix E: Audio, Visual, and Somatosensory Stimulation Information
Appendix F: Consent for Treatment
Appendix G: What I Tell the Client
Appendix H: ClinicalQ Intake Data Form
Appendix I: International 10–20 EEG site locations
Appendix J: Drug Effects on Assessment and Treatment

Appendix A: *ClinicalQ*

Data Required (Amplitude in Microvolts)

Location Cz At this location, record 3–7 Hz, 8–12 Hz, and 16–25 Hz. The recording must be in a continuous sequence to obtain transitions from Eyes-Open (EO) to Eyes-Closed (EC) conditions. The sequence is indicated below with ten 15-s epochs.

P.G. Swingle, *Adding Neurotherapy to Your Practice*,
DOI 10.1007/978-3-319-15527-2

DO NOT pause between epochs. Epochs 9 and 10 are reserved for testing the immediate effects of UnConditioned Stimuli (UCS) or therapeutic sound (harmonics) products for use with braindriving or for clients' home use.

Epoch	@Cz
1	EO
2	EO
3	EC
4	EO
5	(READ)
6	OR
7	(COUNT)
8	EO
9	(TEST)
10	(Harmonic or UCS)

Location O1 At this location, record 3–7 Hz, 8–12 Hz, and 16–25 Hz. The recording must be in a continuous sequence to obtain transitions from Eyes-Open (EO) to Eyes-Closed (EC) conditions. The sequence is indicated below with ten 15-s epochs. DO NOT pause between epochs.

Epoch	@O1
1	EO
2	EO
3	EC
4	EO

Locations F3 and F4 At these locations, record 3–7 Hz, 8–12 Hz, and 16–25 Hz. All recordings are eyes-closed.

Location Fz At this location, record 1.5–2.5 Hz, 3–7 Hz, 8–9 Hz, 11–12 Hz, 8–12 Hz, 16–25 Hz, and 28–40 Hz. All recordings are eyes-closed.

Technical Notes

1. Right ear ground and left ear reference.
2. Epoch length 15 s, shorter if necessary.
3. Recording @ Cz is one continuous run of 10 epochs.
4. Recording @ O1, F4, and F3 is usually in one interrupted run changing electrode position as necessary by pausing data collection.
5. Cognitive challenge is either reading or counting.

6. Data are mean amplitudes.
7. Band amplitudes calculated as square root of single Hz components squared.
8. Unremarkable ranges, listed below, are normative guidelines; specific ranges may vary somewhat based on equipment, environmental conditions, and certainly age of client.
9. The ClinicalQ is *not* appropriate for assessment of stroke, seizure disorders, and traumatic brain injury. ClinicalQ is often appropriate for first assessment of autistic spectrum and brain dysfunction to determine initial treatment protocols to be followed by full QEEG.

Unremarkable Clinical Ranges

1. @Cz: mean Theta/Beta < 2.2; Alpha increase EC > 30 %; Theta/Beta ratio cognitive challenge < 2.2, but no marked difference from mean and Beta increase <20 %; sum of all mean amplitudes, Total Amplitude (TA) < 60.0.
2. @O1: EO and EC Theta/Beta 1.80–2.20; Alpha increase EC > 50 %.
3. @F4 and F3: F4 = F3 in all bands, Theta/Beta ratios <2.00; Theta/Alpha ratio 1.25–1.60; TA = and <60.
4. @Fz: 2 Hz < 9.0; 28–40/Beta 0.45–0.55; 28–40 and Beta < 15.0; 8–9/11–12 < 1.5.

Clinical Implications of Remarkable Ranges

The following clinical probes should be considered as suggestions for developing a behavioral profile of the client. Remarkable ranges do not validate a clinical diagnosis. Similar remarkable patterns can be associated with different clinical profiles. For example, developmental delay, fetal alcohol syndrome, and some autistic spectrum profiles can have very similar remarkable EEG patterns. It is important to keep in mind, therefore, that the remarkable ranges indicate behavioral inefficiencies and not necessarily clinical diagnoses. Unique remarkable patterns are associated with some specific conditions, such as Common Attention Deficit Disorder (CADD) (item 1 under Cz, with no other remarkable ranges). It is the treatment specificity afforded by identifying remarkable ranges rather than diagnostic labeling that makes the ClinicalQ a valuable rapid intake procedure. The following suggested clinical probes are not exhaustive. As the data presented in this book indicate, the qualitative features and specifics of the client's condition can be greatly enhanced by careful analyses and consideration of the combinations of neurological features of the ClinicalQ. The experienced clinician will identify many patterns associated with specific client complaints.

Basic clinical probes for location Cz

Formula Amplitude in microvolts (μv)	Norms	Remarkable range	Clinical implication probe
Alpha response			
Alpha(EC) – Alpha(EO)/Alpha(EO)	>30 %	<30 % or negative	If <30 % or negative, ask about visual processing (memory) problem; poor retention of information and/or poor short-term memory; exposure to severe emotional stressor; also refer to O1 Alpha Response % change
Alpha recovery			
Alpha(EO) before – Alpha(EO) after/Alpha(EO) before	<25 %	>25 %	If >25 %, ask about foggy thinking; older clients ask about cognitive decline, sleep problems, and medications; younger clients probe sleep deprivation, marijuana
Theta(EC)/SMR(EC)	<3.0	>3.0	If >3.0, ask about inability to sit still or quiet the body; sleep disturbance as in trouble falling asleep If >3.0, ask about problems related to muscle activity such as headaches, chronic pain, body tremors, dystonia, and seizure disorders that have a motor component
Theta(EO)/Beta(EO)	<2.2	>2.2	If >2.2, ask about CADD to see if focus and attention are a problem; also refer to T/B (UT) description
Theta(UT)/Beta(UT)	<2.2	>2.2	If >2.2, ask about CADD; ratio should drop under task when compared to eyes open If >2.2 and if Theta(EO)/Beta(EO) < 2.2, ask about ADD and/or problems with poor reading comprehension/retention and getting tired when reading
		>3.0	If >3.0, ask about ADHD
Beta(EO) – Beta(UT)/Beta(EO)	<15 %	>15 %	If >15 %, ask about getting overly tired when reading or problem solving
T/B (EO) – T/B (UT)/T/B(EO)	<15 %	>15 %	If >15 %, ask about CADD
Theta Omni % change			
Theta(Omni) – Theta(EO)/ Theta(EO)	<–5.0 %	Positive %	If Positive %, Theta increased with Omni sound, do not prescribe for home use If <–5.0 % with Omni sound, prescribe for home use
Total amplitude (EC)			
Theta(EC) + Alpha(EC) + Beta(EC)	<60	>60	If >60, ask about development delay, autistic spectrum behavior, marked cognitive deficits
Peak alpha frequency (EC)	>9.5	<9.5	If <9.5, ask about mental sluggishness
Peak alpha frequency (EO)	>9.5	<9.5	If <9.5, ask about mental sluggishness

Basic clinical probes for location O1

Formula Amplitude in microvolts (μv)	Norms	Remarkable range	Clinical implication probe
Alpha response			
Alpha(EC) – Alpha(EO)/Alpha(EO)	>50 %	<50 % or negative	If <50 % or negative, ask about traumatic stress (see also response at Cz), poor retention of information If 150 % +, ask about artistic interest or skills (visual arts, dance, poetry, carpentry, etc.)
Alpha recovery			
Alpha(EO) before – Alpha(EO) after/Alpha(EO) before	<25 %	>25 %	If >25 %, ask about foggy thinking; ask about cognitive decline, sleep problems, medications
Theta(EO)/Beta(EO)	1.8–2.2	<1.8	If <1.8, ask about poor stress tolerance, racing thoughts, anxiety, inefficient self-quieting, sleep problems, symptoms of depression
		≪1.8	If ≪1.8, ask about predisposition to self-medicating behaviors (e.g., alcohol problem), GAD, and stress-precipitated depression
		>3.0	If >3.0, ask about cognitive deficiencies or Asperger's patterns; also see F4/F3 Beta for symptoms. Also applies to T/B (EC), below
Theta(EC)/Beta(EC)	1.8–2.2	<1.5	If about = or <1.5, ask about sleep disturbance. See Theta/Beta (EO), above, for description of probes
T/B(EO) – T/B(EC)/T/B(EO)	> –25 %	< –25 %	If negative and < –25 %, question about sleep-onset difficulties If % is positive, indicates an increase from EO to EC
Total amplitude (EC)			
Theta(EC) + Alpha(EC) + Beta(EC)	<60	>60	If >60, ask about development delay, autistic spectrum behavior, marked cognitive deficits
Peak alpha frequency (EC)	>9.5	<9.5	If <9.5, ask about mental sluggishness
Peak alpha frequency (EO)	>9.5	<9.5	If <9.5, ask about mental sluggishness

Basic clinical probes for locations F3 and/or F4

Formula Amplitude in microvolts (μv)	Norms	Remarkable range	Clinical implication probe
Theta(EC)/Beta(EC)	<2.2	>2.2	If >2.2, ask about cognitive deficiencies associated with retrieval of information, impulse control, emotional volatility, etc. Ask about depression in adults and impulse control in children
Theta(EC)/Alpha(EC)	1.2–1.6	<1.0	If <1.0, ask about frontal Alpha ADD—problems with organization, sequencing, sustained focus, planning, task completion, staying on task, talkativeness
		≪0.8	If ≪0.8, ask about fibromyalgia, chronic fatigue, and sleep disturbance
Total amplitude (EC)			
Theta(EC) + Alpha(EC) + Beta(EC)	<60	>60	If >60, ask about development delays, autism spectrum disorder (especially if O1 Theta is high and the anterior cingulate gyrus is "hot"); memory/cognitive deficits in adults

Basic clinical probes for locations Fz

Fz Amplitude in microvolts (μv)	Norms	Remarkable range	Clinical implication probe
Delta (EC)	<9.0	>9.0	If >9.0, ask about cognitive deficits such as problems with concentration, forgetfulness, and comprehension Higher values can be associated with developmental delays and pain; will usually see remarkable patterns in F3 and F4 if Delta is high
HiBeta/Beta (EC)	0.45–0.55	<0.45	If <0.45, ask about passiveness
		>0.55	If >0.55, ask about stubborn behavior, OC tendencies or OCD, perseveration in autistic spectrum behaviors. Assume hot midline (anterior cingulate gyrus) in treatment of autistic spectrum behaviors
		>0.60 <0.40	If >0.60 or <0.40, ask about anxiety
		>0.80	If >0.80, ask about O/C behaviors
		<0.35	If <0.35, problematic passivity
			Caution! If there is extremely elevated Beta, minimal ratio may result that does not indicate passive behavior
Sum HiBeta + Beta	<15	>15	If >15, ask about autistic spectrum behavior. Implications of 2 above ratios apply only if sum of amplitudes of HiBeta + Beta <15 If >15, but HiBeta/Beta is within normative range, ask about fretting and assume hot midline in treatment of autistic spectrum behaviors
		>15	If >15, "hot" midline
LoAlpha(EC)/HiAlpha(EC)	<1.5	>1.5	If >1.5, ask about cognitive inefficiency, age-related deficits in memory and cognitive processing, and sleep If >1.5, ask about problems with concentration and forgetfulness
		≫1.5	If ≫ 1.5, ask about developmental delays, marked cognitive deficits The lower this ratio, the better, as it reflects more efficient brain functioning
Peak frequency alpha (EC)	>9.5	<9.5	If <9.5 ask about mental sluggishness

Appendix B: Bloodless Brain Surgery (Brainwave Biofeedback and Neurotherapy)

I cannot claim that the title "Bloodless Brain Surgery" was my idea. It was suggested by a client who experienced a marked reduction in symptoms that had remained unchanged after many years of other treatments, both medical and alternative. Brainwave modification treatment is not new and it is really quite simple. Brainwaves (the EEG) are electrical signals from the brain that can be measured from the surface of the skull. These brainwaves indicate how the brain is functioning. When we sleep the brain produces more slow activity such as DELTA waves (0.5–2 cycles per second or Hertz [Hz]). When we daydream the brain produces more Theta activity (4–7 Hz). Concentration results in greater Beta activity (16–25 Hz).

Everything would be fine if Delta is high when we sleep, Theta high when we daydream, and Beta dominant when we are paying attention to a lecture. However, if the brain produces high amplitude Theta when we are trying to concentrate, then we have a problem, and this is precisely the problem that children with some forms of Attention Deficit Disorder (ADD) experience. Their brains are producing wave forms associated with daydreaming or light sleep when they are trying their best to concentrate. One way of dealing with this problem is to give the child drugs that stimulate the central nervous system. A better way to fix the problem is by teaching the child to correct brainwave activity. How do we do that? Simple! We let the child play a type of video game but only with the brain. When the brain is doing what we want, such as reduce the amount of Theta activity, then balloons move on the computer monitor or a clown-like figure stays out of water. With older children and adults, we often simply have a tone signal when the brain is producing the waves that we want.

The landmark breakthroughs in the field of clinical psychoneurophysiology (the treatment of conditions by focusing on both psychological and physiological causes) occurred decades ago. One such breakthrough was when Dr. Miller at Yale University demonstrated that rats could control their heart rates; the second was when Dr. Sterman at UCLA showed that cats could control their brainwaves. Just imagine if people can control physiological functions such as heart rate and brain activity, then they should be able to correct conditions associated with those functions. Dr. Sterman made another remarkable discovery. He found that cats that have learned to increase a specific brainwave were resistant to induced seizures, "Voila," the brainwave treatment for epilepsy and other seizure disorders, was born.

The field of brainwave modification therapy or neurotherapy has experienced explosive growth. We can now do full brain maps as a simple in-office procedure to diagnose many troubling conditions. For mild traumatic brain injury, we look for the location of the damage and specifically treat the problems of body pain, mood disorder, concentration, memory, fine motor skills, sleep, and articulation.

Many troubling conditions have definite brainwave patterns. Genetically predisposed alcoholics (and other addictions) are often deficient in Theta amplitude in the back of the brain. The different forms of ADD and ADD with hyperactivity (ADHD) have patterns such as too much Theta activity on the top of the head, too much

8–12 Hz activity over the front part of the brain, or too little Theta activity in the back of the brain. Post-accident fibromyalgia is often associated with too much slow activity over the front of the brain. Depression is often associated with too much activity over the right front part of the brain. Many persons suffering from Postraumatic Stress Disorder (PTSD) have deficiencies in slow-wave amplitude in the back of the brain and a deficient increase in a particular wave band when they close their eyes. As you will note from the above list, some of these problems are genetic in nature, others reflect brain injury, and others are associated with psychological trauma. The remarkable feature of brain wave modification therapies is that the origin of the problem seems of limited importance. Genetic predispositions can be fixed as can the result of emotional trauma.

Sometimes the EEG does not show any obvious abnormalities even though the client has serious symptoms. This situation is often found with seizure disorders in which the person experiences serious seizures, but no EEG abnormalities can be detected even during the seizure. We know from the work of Dr. Sterman that we can markedly reduce seizure episodes by increasing 13–15 Hz amplitude over a particular brain location.

Sometimes when working with a client with several problems, we have to be extremely precise in increasing the amplitude of one brainwave in a specific area but decreasing the amplitude of that same wave in an adjoining brain area. Such a situation is found when working with adult clients who are both alcoholic and suffer from ADD. We want more Theta activity in the back of the brain but less Theta activity at the top of the head. Clearly, one wants only highly trained professionals to administer these treatments.

Appendix C: Child Intake Questionnaire

Child Form

To be completed by Parent/Guardian

______________________________	______________________________
Child's name	Parent/Guardian

The following items will help to quantify some of the important issues and concerns related to your child's treatment. Please provide your best estimate of how you think your child is now. Indicate your assessment by assigning a number from 1 to 5 according to the following scale:

5 = Very true
4 = Mostly true
3 = Somewhat true
2 = Rarely true
1 = Not true

1. ______ Easy to anger
2. ______ Stubborn
3. ______ Sleep Disturbances
4. ______ Hyperactive
5. ______ Easily frightened
6. ______ Artistic
7. ______ Talkative
8. ______ Forgetful
9. ______ Attention problems in school
10. ______ Obsessive
11. ______ Problems with retention
12. ______ Unhappy
13. ______ Indifferent
14. ______ Poor self-esteem
15. ______ Defiant
16. ______ Too willing to please
17. ______ Frequently ill
18. ______ Anxious
19. ______ Aggressive
20. ______ Unresponsive to other's feeling

Appendix D: Adult Intake Questionnaire

Name:________________________________ Date:_________

The following brief questionnaire will help to quantify some of the important issues and concerns related to your treatment. Please provide your best estimate of how you think you are now. Indicate your answers to the questions by assigning a number from 1 to 5 according to the following scale:

5 = Very true of me
4 = Mostly true of me
3 = Somewhat true of me
2 = Rarely true of me
1 = Not true of me

1. ______ I get angry easily.
2. ______ I am stubborn.
3. ______ I feel depressed.
4. ______ I am very anxious.
5. ______ I am very artistic.
6. ______ I feel tired and fatigued.
7. ______ I check things I know I have already done.
8. ______ I do things I do not want to do because I cannot resist doing them.
9. ______ I feel tired and fatigued much of the time.

10. ______ I am a perfectionist.
11. ______ I am too willing to please others.
12. ______ People like me.
13. ______ I am easily frightened.
14. ______ Sometimes I cannot get rid of annoying or disturbing thoughts.
15. ______ I laugh a lot.
16. ______ I fly off the handle.
17. ______ I feel worthless.
18. ______ In disagreements it is my way or no way.
19. ______ I do not have much to look forward to.
20. ______ I find it hard to concentrate.
21. ______ I often do not remember what I have just read.
22. ______ I am forgetful.
23. ______ I am physically unwell.
24. ______ I have a positive emotional life.
25. ______ I have sleep problems.
26. ______ I feel restless and cannot sit still.
27. ______ I am easily annoyed or irritated

Appendix E: Audio, Visual, and Somatosensory Stimulation

Audio, visual, and somatosensory stimulation are frequently used in neurotherapy. The uses of these stimulation procedures are explained to clients in the intake assessment session. Stimulation is used to increase the efficacy of treatment and thereby markedly reduce the number of sessions required for treating many disorders. Usually some form of stimulation is provided for the client to self-administer at home. Such home-based procedures include self-administered tapping of specific points on the body, audio stimulation, audiovisual stimulation delivered by a light and sound device with stimulation goggles and headsets, and micro-amperage stimulators to deliver weak electrical stimulation to specific points on the body.

Audio Stimulation In neurotherapy, the audio stimulation used, either in office or at home, is usually a harmonic that is embedded in a filtered "pink noise," a sound like the whooshing of an air conditioner. Considerable research has explored the effects of these harmonics on brain activity. Because these harmonics have specific effects on brainwave activity, they are often used to potentiate desired brainwave changes. Some of these harmonics have a calming effect, whereas others are designed to increase focus and alertness. In office, these harmonics are often used to enhance the brainwave changes the client is attempting to accomplish in a neurotherapy session, such as brainwave biofeedback. Harmonics are frequently used when treating autistic or delayed children to calm the child so that neurotherapy may proceed. In office, the harmonics or other therapeutic sounds are usually delivered with headsets so only the client under treatment is affected. In the home environment, the sounds are often delivered "open air" with loudspeakers. Persons not under treatment may be affected by these sounds, so care should be taken to minimize exposure of other persons in the acoustic environment. Most of these therapeutic sounds will not adversely affect others, but some sounds do have stimulating properties which could be uncomfortable for those not under treatment. The harmonics used in neurotherapy have been designed to be used at very low intensity. If you experience discomfort, either in office or at home, it is probably the result of setting the volume too high. Similarly, if you experience no satisfactory effect of the stimulation after prolonged use, the volume is probably too high and outside the window of effectiveness.

Visual Stimulation Visual stimulation is frequently used in neurotherapy and occasionally portable units are provided for clients to use at home. We have found that visual stimulation and feedback used in neurotherapy can be remarkably effective in the treatment of autism and many learning disorders. In such cases, the visual stimulation is presented with small lights mounted on eyeglass frames around the child's field of vision. The child can see through the stimulating field, so is able to read, see, and communicate with the therapist, draw, or do mathematical problems and the like, while being visually stimulated. Another light source that is often used in such cases is a stand-alone light strobe. This is a gooseneck type of fixture with small lights that is directed at material the child is reading. Often these stand-alone fixtures are used for severely hyperactive autistic children who have not yet been able to wear the eyeglasses.

Visual stimulation is also used in the neurotherapeutic treatment of many other disorders including attention deficiencies, dementia, addictions, sleep disorders, alcoholism, chronic pain, chronic fatigue, depression, and traumatic stress disorders. The light stimulation used in such cases, particularly with adults, is delivered with closed eyeglasses with light emitting diodes surrounding the eyes, which are kept closed during treatment. Depending on the treatment, the light stimulation frequency can be calming or arousing, or various combinations of frequencies.

Feelings of agitation and/or headache are occasionally reported. These discomforts are associated with stimulation that is too intense. These side effects are self-limiting in that reduced stimulation usually eliminates the discomfort. Stimulation intensity can be reduced by lowering the brightness or changing the color of the lights. Clients usually self-adjust the light intensity and often mistakenly assume that more intense stimulation is more beneficial. Brightness should always be adjusted to a comfortable level. In fact, there is considerable evidence indicating that very low intensity stimulation may be much more effective than high intensity stimulation.

About 5 % of people with epilepsy are photosensitive and prone to seizure when exposed to light stimulation. At intake, clients are screened for seizure and traumatic brain injury histories. Portable light stimulation devices are never provided for home use if clients report seizure or head injury histories. In office, there are occasions when such stimulation procedures might be used if such use seems therapeutically appropriate and the client is prepared to proceed, even with a seizure history. Generally, however, light stimulation is never suggested for persons with histories that would indicate seizure risk.

Photosensitivity seizure in the general non-epileptic adult population is extremely rare. About one in 20,000 adults, with no seizure history, has photosensitivity. Most photosensitive individuals experience their first seizure while watching television and about 75 % experience their first seizure before the age of 20. Photosensitivity in children with no seizure history is somewhat higher, until the age of about 20, when about 75 % of photosensitive individuals will have been identified after having a seizure. Visual stimulation is used in most of the neurotherapy sessions to potentiate brain wave changes and to mitigate boredom with children. Should a parent be concerned, the visual component can be eliminated, although the occurrence of photosensitivity, even in children, is rare. The treatment of autistic and delayed children relies very heavily on visual stimulation procedures. Similarly, teaching children to read or spell, or to improve these skills, likewise relies extensively on visual stimulation procedures. The risk of photosensitive seizures in children without seizure history would be about 1 in 4,000. One should also keep in mind that if a child is photosensitive, they will likely have a seizure at some time before the age of 20, and having a first seizure in a therapeutic environment is certainly safer than many other locations. Identifying a child with photosensitive epilepsy can be beneficial in that precautions can be taken to prevent seizures in other, less safe, environments. Having a first seizure does not make future seizures more likely. These risk factors do not apply, of course, to the seizure-disordered client. The treatment of seizure disorders does not involve visual stimulation. However, seizure-disordered clients under treatment for severe learning problems may elect to accept the higher seizure risk to facilitate treatment.

Parents, guardians, or other persons accompanying the client in the treatment room should remember that when visual stimulation is delivered, either with a stand-alone strobe or open eyeglasses, their own seizure history may be relevant. Although the risk is trivial, observers with a history of seizures should orient themselves away from the visual stimulation being delivered to the client.

Somatosensory and Cranial Stimulation Somatosensory stimulation is usually self-administered by tapping or rubbing specific points on the body. There are some points on the body that when stimulated result in measurable changes in brain wave activity. These stimulation protocols are often used with neurotherapy in the treatment of phobias and seizure disorders. These body stimulation procedures are frequently used together with harmonic stimulation. Somatosensory stimulation can also be applied with micro-amperage electrical stimulation. As with manual stimulation, micro-amperage stimulation of specific points on the body has been found to have measurable effects on brain activity. Often used to enhance body quiescence during neurotherapy, the level of stimulation should always be below the client's feeling threshold.

Cranial micro-amperage stimulation is usually applied to the ear lobes or on the mastoid process behind the ears. Occasionally used in office, cranial stimulators are usually provided for the client to use at home. Cranial micro-amperage stimulation is a very effective therapy for the treatment of anxiety disorders, depression, addictions such as alcoholism, chronic pain, and sleep disturbance. The cranial stimulators prescribed for home use are Class IIa, Type B medical devices as classified by the Federal Drug Administration (USA). In the USA, a prescription is required from a licensed healthcare practitioner, but these devices are available in Canada without prescription. Feelings of agitation or headache are occasionally reported. These side effects are usually the result of stimulation that is too strong. The stimulation should always be below feeling threshold. When applied in this correct manner, side effects such as headache are very rare. Although completely safe, we never prescribe cranial or somatosensory electrical stimulation for use with children.

Appendix F: Consent for Treatment

I have read the information on the stimulation procedures. I hereby freely and voluntarily agree to have the following stimulation procedures used with me as part of my treatment.

Visual stimulation	Yes	No
Audio stimulation	Yes	No
Micro-amperage stimulation	Yes	No

____________________ ____________________

Signed Date

Appendix G: What I Tell the Client

The thrust of my comments to clients is always that neurotherapy is a naturalistic and safe procedure that is a learning process. Even though the equipment used in neurofeedback and the database used for diagnostic purposes are FDA(US) registered and compliant, I nonetheless structure my remarks to clients in a manner that depathologizes both their condition and the treatment procedures. Clients are told that they will learn how to nudge their brain into more normative functioning ranges. I further describe optimal functioning or peak performance training as an extension of neurotherapy. I point out that many professional athletes do neurotherapy to strengthen their skills (at this point I usually make reference to the Italian soccer team that won the 2006 World Cup in which the entire team received neurotherapy). I might also comment that the optimizing procedures are often used by professional performing artists, CEOs of large companies, and elite military.

Introduction

"Do you know what I do?" (if the client offers an opinion I attempt to make a positive extension of their comment).

"What I do is look at the way the brain functions."

"I'm looking for areas of inefficiency in the way the brain functions." "Those areas where the brain is not functioning efficiently are associated with various symptoms and problems that have brought you here today."

“If we find areas of inefficiency, the way the areas are corrected is called neurotherapy.” “There are three general types of treatment in neurotherapy.” “The first is neurofeedback, or brainwave biofeedback.” “This is the form of treatment that most people have heard about.” “For neurofeedback we measure a particular aspect of brain functioning and when the brain is doing what we want, that is, when it is moving toward greater efficiency, you will hear a tone and/or see something move on the computer monitor.” “The feedback is telling you about a brain activity that you can’t feel but you make use of that information to learn how to self-regulate brain wave activity.”

“The second type of treatment is the braindrivers.” In braindriving, we measure a specific brain activity and based on that measurement we stimulate with lights, sound, micro-amperage stimulation, electromagnetic stimulation, and the like. The system is a closed loop in the sense that the stimulation changes on a moment-to-moment basis depending on the activity of the brain. The purpose of this procedure is to nudge the brain into more normative functioning.”

“The third class of treatments is those that you administer to yourself at home. This could include relaxation exercises, light and sound stimulation, cranial electrical stimulators, and the like. We prescribe these devices and procedures because we know that they influence brain wave activity in a particular way; we know because we test the effects of these devices on the brain activity of each client to determine precisely the effect they will have on the client’s brain functioning.”

“I’m going to put a wire on each of your ears and one on top of your head that I will move around. You won’t feel anything as this is measurement only. I will ask you to open and close your eyes, read something for a brief period, and I’m going to play a sound that sounds like “shush.” After I record the data, I will do a few calculations and then go over the results with you in detail to determine if what the brain is telling me is consistent with your personal experience. Then we will figure out what form of treatments we can use to correct the problems.”

“As I said, you will not feel anything this is measurement only. You will see the electrical activity of your brain on the computer monitor. Please place both feet flat on the floor and don’t move too much since the system is movement sensitive. At the end, I will do some calculations and go over the results in very great detail.”

Introduction with Children

Children are often nervous and frightened when they first enter the office. I usually start by saying that “I’m going to set you up like an astronaut. Astronauts usually have wires on them while they are flying their spacecraft so people on the ground can see how they are doing. I am going to put a wire on each of your ears and one on top of your head to measure the electricity coming from your brain. Did you know that your brain produces electricity? And NOTHING hurts. I’m just going to measure the electricity coming from your head just like an astronaut. Do you play any sports? Well lots of professional athletes do this and lots of singers and actors as well. Are you a collector? Well when you are through today, you can look in Dr. Swingle's Treasure Chest. The Treasure Chest contains coins from all over the world, semiprecious stones like jade, and fossils like real dinosaur bones and shark's teeth and you can take one for yourself. Sound like a deal?" (The Treasure Chest contains educational items like fossils, coins, paper money, semiprecious stones, and the like but no toys or candy or plastic trinkets. On the wall above the chest are charts, maps, and information sheets to help the child identify the item, its age, location, and the like. Since the child's brain is alert after treatment, they retain the information about the item and often dazzle their teachers at show-and-tell with their breadth of knowledge about these interesting items).

Joking with the child and keeping everything light is very important. I DO NOT allow the parent to tell me the child's problems at this time so the child is exposed to a very unique experience that is very different from what they expect. They usually expect to hear their parents tell the tale of woe about the child's "challenges" and often how long suffering and patient they have been in caring for this child. When I first put on the electrodes, if the child is young and nervous I will ask the child to hold various items such as the cotton ball or the cotton-tipped swab. I tell the child often that "nothing hurts" and let them know that the alcohol on the ear lobe will feel cold—sometimes I will touch their arm with the alcohol pad to let them feel the chill. When I scratch the head for the electrode placement I often say "Ouch!"—Inevitably the child laughs and says that it doesn't hurt. If the child does complain I usually say "phooey, that doesn't hurt."

Explaining the Data

After the data are collected, I do the calculations and record the results on the data sheet shown in Appendix I. I make a copy of the data summary sheet and the electrode placement schematic and give them to the client. I also give the client a pad of paper and a pen and make the statement "if you want to make any notes." Whenever possible I give these items directly to the client. For example, the client may be a child of 12 so I give the child the items directly and ask the parents to gather around so we can go over the results. I still have not allowed the parent to tell the tale of woe and the child usually feels strongly engaged in this process. I do this to again give the child the strong impression that this is a very unique experience and that they are an integral part of the process of correcting their problems.

Pointing to the locations on the schematic "We had a look at five critical areas in the brain. Cz is directly over the sensory motor cortex, an area of the brain that is involved in movement and processing of sensory information. O1, back of the brain, is an area associated with calming the brain. And then we looked right across the frontal strip. F3 is the left frontal cortex, F4 is the right, and Fz is right on the frontal midline. As you know the frontal regions of the brain are implicated in everything including cognitive, intellectual activity, and emotional regulation.

"We looked at many different brainwaves ranging from very slow Delta waves at 2 cycles per second to very fast Gamma waves at 40 cycles per second. For example, Theta brainwaves are between 3 and 7 cycles per second and are considered slow waves. The significance of the Theta brain activity depends on brain location. In some areas, high amplitude Theta is associated with hypoactivity, daydreaming, mind wandering, early sleep, or drowsiness. In other areas of the brain, strong Theta can be an indicator of inefficiency of brain function. In some areas of the brain, one wants to see a lot of Theta activity. Theta in these regions is associated with the brain's ability to calm itself. Experienced meditators, for example, are increasing Theta amplitude in specific areas of the brain when they meditate. So it all depends on just where the Theta activity is in the brain."

"Alpha is brain activity between 8 and 12 cycles per second. Alpha is an extraordinarily important brainwave for diagnostic purposes. It tells us about brain efficiency, it tells us about visualization skills, it tells us about emotional trauma, and it is the idling frequency in the brain. When we are training the brain for optimal or peak performance, we work a lot with the Alpha activity. As we get older our Alpha slows down so for the elderly we keep Alpha fast to prevent dementias, delay Alzheimer's, and strengthen immune functioning."

"Finally Beta is brainwave activity between 16 and 25 cycles per second. Beta is strong when the brain is processing information. When you focus your attention, for example, Beta will become stronger in some areas of the brain."

"Now the electrode that I use is sitting over about 100,000 brain cells and each one of those is firing multiple times per second so these numbers are associated with a lot of brain activity. We assess brain efficiency by looking at the ratios among various brainwave bands and the changes in brainwave activity that take place in different states such as between eyes-open and eyes-closed conditions or when you are reading. Although we get changes in brainwave amplitude as a function of time of day, your physical condition, your food intake such as caffeinated beverages, medication use, and the like, the ratios and state changes are very robust across these conditions so our diagnostic indicators are stable over multiple recording conditions."

I then proceed to interpret the client's brainwave data as detailed in the suggested probes described in the "Remarkable Ranges" section of Chap. 1. The detail presented above is usually somewhat overwhelming for most clients, but it emphasizes that neurotherapy is a no nonsense, data-driven, objective procedure. It is part of the therapeutic strategy to direct the client to embrace the concept that changing brain activity will change their cognitive and emotional behavior. Clients usually have less of a problem accepting that changing brain activity can result in changes in motor activity such as limited movement resulting from brain injury. However, even in this case, the notion that the brain is plastic and capable of change long after the brain trauma is sometimes difficult because of the misinformation clients receive from our health system. The point, of course, is that at each stage of the intake process of the ClinicalQ, the therapist has the opportunity to help the client to embrace the concepts of neurotherapy and to establish expectations. If, for example, one points out to a client that a particular inefficiency is associated with depression, then the client expects the depression to lift when the inefficiency is corrected.

Appendix H

GENDER:
AGE:

CZ	VALUES
EO Alpha	
EC Alpha	
% Change EO to EC Alpha > 30%	
% Difference EO Alpha from intial EO after EC	
Theta Amplitude EO	
Beta Amplitude EO	
EO Theta/Beta	
Theta Amplitude Under Task (UT)	
Beta Amplitude UT	
UT Theta/Beta	
% Change T/B EO to T/B EO UT	
% UT Beta Increase	
Total Amplitude	
% Change in Theta with Omni	
Theta/SMR EC	

F3 & F4 (ALL EC)	VALUES		% Difference F3-F4
	F3	F4	
Theta/Alpha			
Total Amplitude			
Theta Amplitude			
Alpha Amplitude			
Beta Amplitude			
Theta/Beta			

O1	VALUES
Alpha EO	
Alpha EC	
% Change in Alpha EO to EC	
% Change EO Alpha to EO Alpha after EC	
Theta Amplitude EO	
Beta Amplitude EO	
Theta/Beta EO	
Theta Amplitude EC	
Beta Amplitude EC	
Theta/Beta EC	

FZ (ALL EC)	VALUES
Delta (2Hz)	
HiBeta Amplitude	
Beta Amplitude	
HiBeta/Beta	
Sum HiBeta + Beta	
LoAlpha Amplitude	
HiAlpha Amplitude	
LoAlpha/HiAlpha	
Alpha Peak Frequency	

NOTES FOR F3/F4 DIFFERENCE
F3-F4 / Lowest Amplitude (F3 or F4)
If F4 > F3 Designate +
If F4 < F3 Designate -

Appendix I

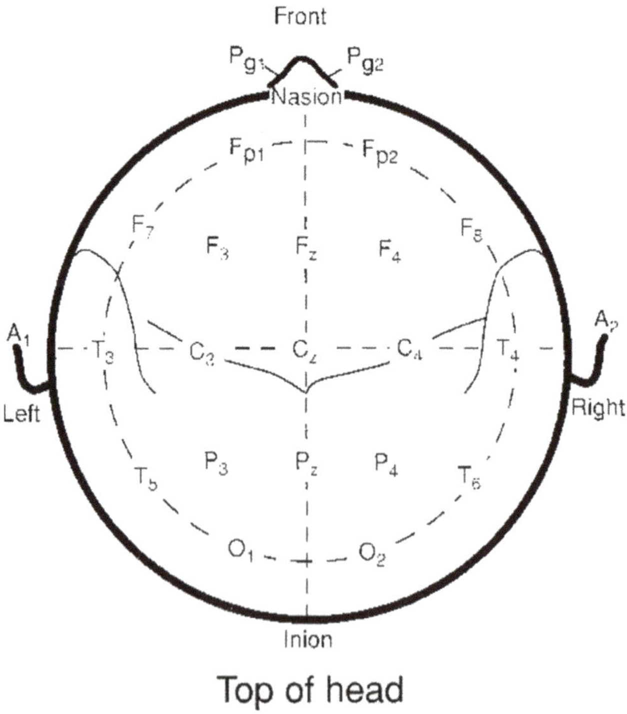

Appendix J: Neurotherapy in Medical Practice

As has been discussed throughout this book, neurotherapy melds perfectly with other treatment metaphors and in particular with psychology and medicine. The following focuses on the interaction between medications and neurotherapy. As is obvious, the amalgamation of these two therapeutic approaches offers substantial benefit to patients.

In general, medications alter amplitudes, but the ClinicalQ ratios are reasonably robust and can be relied upon to guide the development of the clinical treatment protocols. Obviously, drugs that impact narrowly on specific brainwave frequencies will distort the relevant ratios for clinical interpretation. For example, Tetrahydrocannabinol (*THC*), marijuana, increases frontal Alpha which mimics the High Frontal Alpha (HFA) form of ADHD. Interestingly, the behavior of THC-intoxicated individuals also mimics the behavior of the classic HFA adolescent. These behaviors include talkativeness, scattered, social, problems staying on topic, and problems with focus, planning, organizing, and following through on tasks.

The following generalizations can be helpful when interpreting the ClinicalQ with clients who are medicated. They also are relevant when clinicians find that therapeutic progress is slow, indicating that treatment focus may require more aggressive alternatives or efforts to modify medication regimen.

It is also important to keep in mind that medications interact with the client's arousal level, health, and, of course, other medications and chemicals. An under-aroused client, for example, may respond better to neurotherapy when caffeinated but respond poorly to treatment when caffeine consumed when alert. On the other hand, Alpha and Beta are related in the sense that an under-aroused client may respond to treatment with both Alpha and Beta increases. An aroused client may show treatment-specific increases such that Beta increases when Alpha is suppressed. Medications can directly influence treatment therefore by affecting the arousal level of the client.

ClinicalQ assessment data can be very useful for helping physicians to identify medications that have effects on the putative neurological condition associated with the patient's symptoms. The example of the child with diagnosis of ADHD offers a good example of how the intake ClinicalQ data can not only indicate areas for neurotherapeutic treatment but also improve precision of identifying most efficacious medications (see Gunkelman 2014 for discussion of medications for specific forms of ADHD).

Simons and Perlis (2010) suggest the concept of "personalized medicine" to define the process of identifying putative causes for disorders rather than the top-down process of labeling symptoms and then treating the label. As has been discussed at length, this process leads to trial-and-error medicine as well as trial-and-error neurotherapy. It is also in the area of personalized medicine that the blending of neurotherapy with medicine is so efficacious. And the most important concept associated with this positive synergy is that the brain is neurologically plastic.

It is interesting that the Global Genome Study indicated that genetics do not account for much of the statistical variance associated with psychological disorders (Lander 2011). This is the same problem that is associated with normative data bases in the area of neurotherapy. "Normal" are non-symptomatic people. However, as previously discussed, these same individuals may have the same genetic markers as symptomatic people, but they have not manifested to clinical symptom magnitude. This concept of manifested markers is expressed in the term "endophenotype" suggested by Gottesman and Gould (2003) that is essentially a marker when certain heritability markers have been fulfilled.

Increasing efficacy of medication response can be markedly enhanced with ClinicalQ assessment of the patient's neurological state. High frontal Alpha forms of ADHD, for example, do not respond well to medications that are very efficacious for the high central Theta/Beta ratio forms of ADHD. The potential for negative side effects from specific medications may also be identifiable with data from the ClinicalQ.

In addition, some medications may have potential to elicit a patient's neurological predisposition for conditions such as depression, mood volatility, or compulsive behaviors. It is interesting to note that several unusual adverse effects of some dopamine agonist medications may include compulsive gambling, punding, hypersexuality, and overeating (Wolters et al. 2008) even in patients without any prior history of these behaviors (Bostwick et al. 2009).

At the most fundamental level, the data are quite clear that by improving the APF everything works better. As noted below, low APF results in poorer response to many medications including stimulants, antidepressants, and antipsychotics. Even response to rTMS is poorer with slow APF (Arns et al. 2012).

Many psychiatric syndromes are associated with decreased APF including schizophrenia, chronic fatigue syndrome, and hemispheric stroke. With individuals reporting chronic fatigue, APF correlates negatively with self-reported fatigue level (Billiot et al. 1997) as well as an indicator of physical fatigue (Ng and Raveen 2007). Patients with schizophrenia show decreased APF both before and following treatment with an antipsychotic (Canive et al. 1998).

APF has also been found to be related to emotional and autonomic states. Kostyunin and Kulikov (1995) and Kostyunina (1998) found APF increases associated with joy and anger, and APF decreases during fear and sorrow. Clinical individuals are shown to score lower than matched healthy controls on cognitive performance tasks (Klimesch et al. 1990a, b), which supports their reduced cognitive preparedness. There is also a positive correlation between APF and working memory across the age span (Clark et al. 2004).

At the Swingle Clinic, we have found that clients with various forms of cancer who are undergoing some form of treatment including chemotherapy or radiation appear to respond more efficiently when APF is enhanced. These clients are being treated at the clinic not for the cancer but usually for problems such as poor sleep quality and cognitive problems ("chemofog"). However, the limited data do suggest better response with faster APF which is not unexpected given the general beneficial effects on other medication response.

Finally, titration from any chemical has physiological and psychological withdrawal effects. Reduction of stimulants may make a client more agitated because of hypoactivity over the motor cortex or because of reduction of pleasant arousal states. Withdrawal effects can be associated with physiological discomfort or diminished "highs" that have nothing to do with the condition for which the medication was prescribed. That is, a depressed person may experience a physiological angst associated with reduced medication level and misattribute that discomfort to a belief of exacerbation of depression. This is particularly problematic for clients with long histories of severe depression who become terrified of relapse when they experience the physiological response to reduced medication levels.

The following generalizations were derived from Arns (2012), Blume (2006), Gunkelman (2009, 2014), Reeves et al. (1995), and Salinsky et al. (1994, 2002), and data from the Swingle Clinic.

Antidepressants
Increase in slow-frequency amplitude and increase in fast frequency amplitude are most common alterations in the EEG found with these medications. Slowing and/or reduced amplitude of Alpha is also found, more commonly in the older (e.g., amitriptyline) in contrast to newer (e.g., SSRIs) antidepressants. Patients with low APF may not respond effectively to antidepressants (Ulrich et al. 1984).

Anxiolytics
Decrease in Alpha amplitude, mild increase in Theta, and increases in faster Beta amplitude. Often used for clients with seizure disorders as epileptiform activity either decreased or not increased. Benzodiazepines can decrease cerebral blood flow (Forster et al. 1987) with attendant decrease in Alpha Peak Frequency (Clemens et al. 2006). Can cause intoxication like effect "buzz" with patients with elevated frontal Beta amplitude (Porjesz et al. 2002).

Neuroleptics/Antipsychotics
Decreased Beta amplitude, slow Alpha return, increased connectivity, and aperiodic frontal Theta bursts. Increased epileptiform activity. Patients with slow APF may be poor responders to antipsychotics (Itil et al. 1975).

Antiepileptics
Increased Delta and Theta amplitude. Generalized slowing of background EEG. Epileptiform (paroxysmal) prevalence is about 2 % in the general population but about 50–80 % in the ASD populations (Parmeggiani et al. 2010) and about 15–30 % in children diagnosed with ADHD (Arns 2012). Studies have found that anticonvulsants have been effective for ADHD (Davids et al. 2006) and ASD (Yasuhara 2010).

Hormones
Decreased frontal Alpha and increased frontal Beta amplitude. Increase Alpha Peak Frequency. (Early study indicated reduced APF with oral contraceptives.)

Barbiturates
Increased frontal Beta and increased Delta (Roth et al. 1957). Slowing of background EEG at higher doses.

Morphine/Codeine
Increase Alpha amplitude and slowing of Alpha Peak Frequency. May affect (usually increase) REM sleep, hence corrupting sleep assessment EEG.

Alcohol
Slowing of background EEG and rapid increase in Alpha amplitude. May affect (usually increase) Deep Phase sleep, hence corrupting sleep assessment EEG. One of the neurological endotypes found in alcoholics is low Alpha amplitude (Enoch 2003) which is highly heritable (Anokhin 1992) and which is rapidly increased with alcohol consumption. The rapid increase in Alpha amplitude is associated with the addictive property of alcohol for the "genetic" alcoholic.

Nicotine
Temporary increase in Alpha Peak Frequency (APF). Because higher APF is associated with enhanced response to antidepressants, it was hypothesized that for the depressed patients who are nonresponders or poor responders to antidepressants, a Nicotinic Channel Modulator (NCM) may augment clinical response. Research has shown that adjunctive NCM does not augment patient response to either an SSRI or an SNRI (Vieta et al. 2014).

Stimulants
Decreased slow-frequency amplitude, increased Beta amplitude, and increased Alpha amplitude, typically posteriorly with medications such as amphetamine and methylphenidate. Patients with the elevated Theta amplitude and elevated Theta/Beta ratio form of ADHD respond to stimulants (Suffin and Emory 1995). However, those with low Alpha Peak Frequency (APF) often do not respond well to stimulants (Arns et al. 2012). The elevated Theta/Beta ratio can be affected by low Alpha which can be identified on the ClinicalQ either with the Low/High Alpha ratio or APF. Hence, patients with elevated Theta/Beta ratios may respond well to stimulants, but those with Alpha slowing in addition to elevated Theta/Beta ratio, and those with high frontal Alpha amplitude, may not respond well to stimulants.

Interestingly, ADHD children with marked elevation of frontal Beta amplitude often respond to stimulants. This high Beta group also shows symptoms of anxiety, moodiness, and temper problems.

Moderate caffeine, mild Beta increase, and Theta decrease in amplitude. Withdrawal from stimulants including coffee, black teas, and the like: Increased Theta and frontal Alpha amplitude during first few days so initial ClinicalQ should be delayed for about 4 days following withdrawal if possible.

Racetams (like nicotine) increase Alpha Peak Frequency and are used to enhance mental functioning in a wide range of conditions. Also these drugs are used illicitly as "smart drugs" for improving academic performance.

Lithium Carbonate
Increase in Theta and Beta amplitude. Reduction in Alpha amplitude and reduced Alpha response. Increases in epileptiform activity have also been reported.

Conclusions

It is apparent that the addition of neurotherapy to medical practice has substantial benefit. Neurotherapy can aid in the selection as well as the potentiation of medications. As the patient's conditions improve, neurotherapy can effectively guide the rationalization of the pharmaceutical regimen. The target is, of course, the reduction and/or removal of the pharmaceutical agents as the brain functions more efficiently. Research (Monastra et al. 2002) has shown that the combination of medication and neurotherapy can be very efficacious for maintaining improvement in conditions such as ADHD. In the Monastra study, children given both stimulant medication and neurofeedback sustain gains once the medication was removed, whereas the medication only group did not sustain gains once the stimulant was terminated.

Efficient functioning of the brain as it applies to medical treatment focuses on three major components: stress tolerance, depressed mood states, and Alpha Peak Frequency (brain efficiency). Stress tolerance factors are the major contributors to sleep quality problems. As has often been stated, "Fix sleep and everything improves."

Depressed mood has direct effects on immune functioning and in particular on inhibiting activities such as exercise, social engagement, and inquisitiveness that are essential for good emotional as well as physical health. Stable elevated activation of the right frontal cortex, a marker for predisposition to depressed mood states, is associated with lower levels of NK cell activity (Kang et al. 1991). Miller et al. (1999) also report that depression is related to suppression of CD4 count, whereas stress reduction training is related to improve immune functioning (Creswell et al. 2009).

Alpha Peak Frequency is the critical neurological marker for good brain efficiency. When APF is compromised the patient's effective response to virtually the entire array of treatment options is negatively affected. Depressed patients with low APF do not respond as effectively to antidepressants. Increase APF with neurotherapy and the patient will respond more effectively to antidepressants. After stabilization and improved mood state, the patient may be a good candidate for additional neurotherapeutic treatment to further reduce medication levels or to wean off the medication entirely.

Braindriving protocols are particularly useful in general medical practice to quickly quiet patients in high states of angst. Patients who respond well to these more aggressive treatments may be more amenable to reduced pharmaceutical interventions or to elect to try greater self-regulation methods such as home relaxation exercises, neurotherapy, and reduced medication levels or to pursue social support during periods of challenge.

The ClinicalQ can be particularly helpful for assessing the neurological condition of the patient. Patients who report depression symptoms may be "depressed" because of fatigue associated with poor sleep, hopelessness because of debilitating effects of severe anxiety, or cognitive challenges associated with Alpha slowing. Clearly, these patients my respond poorly to antidepressants and more problematically may become chronic because they only appear to respond to sedation to reduce anguish and sleeplessness.

As reviewed throughout this book, neurotherapy has been found to be effective for the treatment of a wide range of disorders. An outcome study on the effects of neurotherapy in a general neurology practice was reported by Koberda et al. (2012).

The 25 patients included in this study presented with a variety of conditions including ADHD, TBI, anxiety, cognitive deficits, autism, seizure disorders, fibromyalgia, depression, Asperger's, pain, tremor, and headache. Of the 25 patients studied, there were an 84 % subjective improvement rate and a 75 % objective improvement in the EEG after completion of the neurotherapeutic treatment.

About the Author

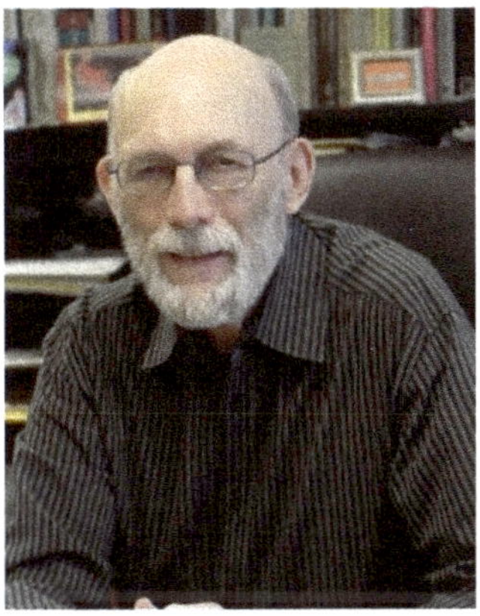

Paul G. Swingle, Ph.D., R.Psych., was Professor of Psychology at the University of Ottawa prior to moving to Vancouver. A Fellow of the Canadian Psychological Association, Dr. Swingle was Lecturer in Psychiatry at Harvard Medical School and during the same time period was Associate Attending Psychologist at McLean Hospital (Boston) where he also was Coordinator of the Clinical Psychophysiology Service. Dr. Swingle was Chairman of the Faculty of Child Psychology at the University of Ottawa and Clinical Supervisor. He has also taught at McGill University, Dalhousie University, and McMaster University. He is a Registered Psychologist in British Columbia and is certified in Biofeedback and Neurotherapy. Since 1997, he has been in private practice in Vancouver, British Columbia, where he founded the Swingle Clinic.

P.G. Swingle, *Adding Neurotherapy to Your Practice*,
DOI 10.1007/978-3-319-15527-2

References

Abstra-Angelakis, E., Stathopoulou, S., Frymiare, J. L., Green, D. L., Lubar, J. F., & Kounios, J. (2007). EEG neurofeedback: A brief overview and an example of peak alpha frequency training for cognitive enhancement in the elderly. *Clinical Neuropsychology, **21***(1), 110–129.

American Heart Association. (2014, June 25). Watching too much TV may increase risk of early death: Three hours a day linked to premature death from any cause. *ScienceDaily*.

Angelakis, E. (2003). Peak alpha frequency: An electroencephalographic measure of cognitive preparedness. *Journal of Neurotherapy, 7*, 27–29 (Abstract).

Anokhin, A. (1992). A genetic study of the human low-voltage electroencephalogram. *Human Genetics, 90*, 99–112.

Anokhin, A. P., Heath, A. C., & Myers, E. (2006). Genetic and environmental influences on frontal EEG asymmetry: A twin study. *Biological Psychiatry, 71*, 289–295.

Arnold, E. M., Goldston, D. B., Ruggiero, A., Reboussin, B. A., Daniel, S. S., & Hickman, E. A. (2003). Rates and predictors of rehospitalisation among formerly hospitalized adolescents. *Psychiatric Services, 54*(7), 994–998.

Arns, M. (2012). EEG-based personalized medicine in ADHD: Individual alpha peak frequency as an endophenotype associated with nonresponse. *Journal of Neurotherapy, 16*, 123–141.

Arns, M., Drinkenburg, W. H. I. M., Fitzgerald, P. B., & Kenemans, J. L. (2012). Neurophysiological predictors of non-response to rTMS in depression. *Brain Stimulation, 5*(4), 569–576.

Arns, M., Gunkelman, J., Olbrich, S., Sander, C., & Hegerl, U. (2010). EEG vigilance and phenotypes in neuropsychiatry: Implications for intervention. In R. Coben & J. Evans (Eds.), *Neuromodulation and neurofeedback: Techniques and applications* (pp. 79–123). New York, NY: Elsevier.

Barry, R. J., Clarke, A. R., McCarthy, R., & Selikowitz, M. (2006). Age and gender effects in EEG coherence: III. *Clinical Neurophysiology, 117*, 243–251.

Basterra-Gortari, F. J., Bes-Rastrollo, M., Gea, A., Núñez-Córdoba, J. M., Toledo, E., & Martínez-González, M. A. (2014). Television viewing, computer use, time driving and all-cause mortality: The SUN Cohort. *Journal of the American Heart Association, 3*, e000864.

Bazanova, O. M., Balioz, N. V., Mauravleva, K. B., & Skoraya, M. V. (2013). Effect of voluntary EEG Alpha power increase training on heart rate variability. *Human Physiology, 39*, 86–97.

Belsky, J., & Pluess, M. (2009). Beyond diathesis stress: Differential susceptibility to environmental influences. *Psychological Bulletin, 135*: 885–908. Doi: 10.1037/a0017376.

Berger, H. (1969). *Hans Berger on the electroencephalograph of man: The fourteen original reports*. Amsterdam: Elsevier.

Biederman, J., Faraone, S., Spencer, T., Mick, E., Monuteaux, M., & Aleardi, M. (2006). Functional impairments in adults with self-reports of diagnosed ADHD. *The Journal of Clinical Psychiatry, 67*, 524–540.

P.G. Swingle, *Adding Neurotherapy to Your Practice*,
DOI 10.1007/978-3-319-15527-2

Budzynski, T., Budzynski, H. K., & Tang, H-Y. (2007). Brain brightening: restoring the aging mind. Chapter in J. R. Evans (Ed.), Handbook of Neurofeedback. Binghampton, NY: Haworth Medical Press, 231–265.

Billiot, K. M., Budzynski, T. H., & Andrasik, F. (1997). EEG patterns and chronic fatigue syndrome. *Journal of Neurotherapy, 2*(2), 20–30.

Bladder, J. C. (2011). Acute inpatient care for psychiatric disorders in the United States, 1966 through 2007. *Achieves of General Psychiatry, 68*(12), 1276–1282.

Blume, W. (2006). Drug effects on EEG. *Journal of Clinical Neurophysiology, 23*, 306–311.

Bostwick, J. M., Hecksel, K. A., Stevens, S. R., Bower, J. H., & Ahlskog, J. E. (2009). Frequency of new-onset pathologic compulsive gambling or hypersexuality after drug treatment of idiopathic Parkinson disease. *Mayo Clinic Proceedings, 84*(4), 310–316.

Boyer, B. A., Bubel, D., Jacobs, S. R., Knolls, M. L., Harwell, V. D., Goscicka, M., et al. (2002). Posttraumatic stress in women with breast cancer and their daughters. *American Journal of Family Therapy, 30*, 323–338.

Boyle, P. A., Barnes, L. L., Buchman, A. S., & Bennet, D. A. (2009). Purpose in life is associated with mortality among community-dwelling older persons. *Psychosomatic Medicine, 71*(5), 574–579.

Bridenbaugh, S. A., & Kressiq, R. W. (2013). Quantitative gait disturbances in older adults with cognitive impairments. *Current Pharmaceutical Design, 20*(19), 3165–3172.

Budzynski, T. (1995, February). *Barebones 14 Hz EEG training for migraine.* Paper presented at the Futurehealth EEG conference, Key West, FL.

Cahn, B. R., & Polich, J. (2006). Meditation states and traits: EEG, ERP, and neuroimaging studies. *Psychological Bulletin, 132*(2), 180–211.

Calvo, A., Moreno, M., Ruiz-Sancho, A., Rapado-Castro, M., & Moreno, C. (2014). Intervention for adolescents with early-onset psychosis and their families: A randomized controlled trial. *Journal of the American Academy of Child and Adolescent Psychiatry, 53*, 688–696.

Canive, J. M., Lewine, J. D., Edgar, J. C., Davis, J. T., Miller, G. A., Torres, F., et al. (1998). Spontaneous brain magnetic activity in schizophrenia patients treated with aripiprazole. *Psychopharmacology Bulletin, 34*(1), 101–105.

Chabot, R. J., diMichele, F., Prichep, L., & John, E. R. (2001). The clinical role of computerized EEG in the evaluation and treatment of learning and attention disorders in children and adolescents. *Journal of Neuropsychiatry and Clinical Neuroscience, 13*, 171–186.

Chabot, R. J., & Sigal, L. H. (1995). QEEG and evoked potentials in the central nervous system Lyme disease. *Clinical Electroencephalography, 26*, 137–145.

Cipriani, A., Furukawa, T. A., Salanti, G., Geddes, J. R., Higgins, J. P., Churchill, R., et al. (2009). Comparative efficiency and acceptability of 12 new-generation antidepressants: A multiple-treatments meta-analysis. *Lancet, 373*, 746–758.

Clark, C. R., Veltmeyer, M. D., Hamilton, R. J., Simms, E., Paul, R., Mermens, D., et al. (2004). Spontaneous alpha peak frequency predicts working memory performance across the age span. *International Journal of Psychophysiology, 53*, 1–9.

Clemens, B., Ménes, A., Piros, P., Bessenyei, M., Altmann, A., Jerney, J., et al. (2006). Quantitative EEG effects of carbamazepine, oxcarbazepine, valproate, lamotrigine, and possible clinical relevance of the findings. *Epilepsy Research, 70*, 190–199.

Colcombe, S. J., Erickson, K. I., Scalf, P. E., Kim, J. S., Prakash, R., McAuley, E., et al. (2006). Aerobic exercise training increases brain volume in aging humans. *Journal of Gerontology, 61A*(11), 1166–1170.

Copeland, W. E., Angold, A., Shanahan, L., & Costello, E. J. (2014). Longitudinal patterns of anxiety from childhood to adulthood: The Great Smoky Mountains Study. *Journal of the American Academy of Child and Adolescent Psychiatry, 53*(1), 21–33.

Creswell, J. D., Myers, H. F., Cole, S. W., & Irwin, M. R. (2009). Mindfulness meditation training effects on CD4+ T lymphocytes in HIV-1 infected adults: A small randomized control trial. *Brain, Behavior and Immunity, 23*, 184–188.

Cummings, C. M., Caporino, N. E., Sttipani, C. A., Read, K. L., Sherrill, J., Walkup, J. T., et al. (2013). The therapeutic relationship in Cognitive-Behavioral Therapy and pharmacology for anxious youth. *Journal of Consulting and Clinical Psychology, 81*(5), 859–864.

Daban, C., & Vieta, E. (2008). Safety and efficacy of Vagus Nerve Stimulation in treatment-resistant depression. A systematic review. *Journal of Affective Disorders, 16*, 1–15.

Davidson, R. J. (1992). Anterior cerebral asymmetry and the nature of emotion. *Brain & Cognition, 20*, 125–151.

Davids, E., Kis, B., Specka, M., & Gastpar, M. (2006). A pilot clinical trial of oxcarbazepine in adults with attention-deficit hyperactivity disorder. *Progress in Neuro-Psychopharmacology and Biological Psychiatry, 30*, 1033–1038.

Dawson, G., Frey, K., Panagiotides, H., Osterling, J., & Hessl, D. (1997). Infants of depressed mothers exhibit atypical frontal brain activity: A replication and extension of previous findings. *Journal of Child Psychology and Psychiatry and Allied Disciplines, 38*(2), 179–186.

DiCara, L. V., & Miller, N. E. (1969). Heart-rate learning in the noncurarized state, transfer to the curarized state, and subsequent retraining in the noncurarized state. *Physiology and Behavior, 4*, 621–624.

Donaldson, M., Donaldson, C. C. S., Mueller, H. H., & Sella, G. (2003). QEEG patterns, psychological status and pain reports of fibromyalgia sufferers. *American Journal of Pain Management, 13*(2), 1–27.

Donaldson, C. C. S., Sella, G. E., & Mueller, H. H. (1998). Fibromyalgia: A retrospective study of 252 consecutive referrals. *Canadian Journal of Clinical Medicine, 5*, 116–127.

Doppelmayr, M., & Klimesch, W. (2003). EEG and intelligence. *Journal of Neurotherapy, 7*, 45–46 (Abstract).

Dougherty, D. D., Baer, L., Cosgrove, G. R., Cassem, E. H., Price, B. H., Nierenberg, A. A., et al. (2002). Prospective long-term follow-up of 44 patients who received cingulotomy for treatment-refractory obsessive-compulsive disorder. *American Journal of Psychiatry, 159*(2), 269–275.

Dupont, F., & Swingle, P. G. (1996, August). *Troubles deficitaires de l'attention et reduction de l'activité cérébrale theta par une technique subliminale auditive.* Paper presented at the International Congress of Psychology, Montreal, Quebec.

Gruber, B.L., and Taub, E. (1998) Thermal and EMG biofeedback learning in nonhuman primates. *Applied Psychophysiology and Biofeedback, 23*, 1–12.

Gunkelman, J. (2006) Transcend the DSM using phenotypes. *Biofeedback, 34*, 95–98.

Enoch, M. A. (2003). Genetics of alcoholism using intermediate phenotypes. *Alcoholism: Clinical and Experimental Research, 27*, 776–787.

Fiocco, A. J., Shatenstein, B., Guylaine, F., Payette, H., Belleville, S., Kergoat, M., et al. (2012). Sodium intake and physical activity impact cognitive maintenance in order adults: The NuAge study. *Neurobiology of Aging, 33*(4), 821–829.

Foulds, J., McSorley, K., Sneddon, J., Feyeraend, C., Jarvis, M. J., & Russell, M. A. (1994). Effect of subcutaneous nicotine injections of EEG alpha frequency in non-smokers: A placebo-controlled pilot study. *Psychopharmacology, 115*(1–2), 163–166.

Forster A, Juge O, Louis M, Nahory A. (1987) Effects of a specific benzodiazepine antagonist (RO 15–1788) on cerebral blood flow. *Anesthesiology and Analgesia. 66*(4), 309–313.

Frederick, J. A., DeAnna, L., Timmermann, D. L., Russell, H. L., & Lubar, J. F. (2005). EEG coherence effects of audio-visual stimulation (AVS) at dominant and twice dominant alpha frequency. *Journal of Neurotherapy, 8*(4), 25–42.

Ginsburg, G. S., Becker, E. M., Keeton, C. P., Sakolsky, D., Piacentini, J., Albano, A. M., et al. (2014). Naturalistic follow-up of youths treated for pediatric anxiety disorders. *Journal of the American Medical Association Psychiatry, 71*(3), 310–318.

Goodman, D. (2007). The consequences of Attention-Deficit/Hyperactivity Disorder in adults. *Journal of Psychiatric Practice, 13*, 318–327.

Gottesman, I. I. & Gould, T. D. (2003). The endophenotype concept in psychiatry: Etymology and strategic intentions. *American Journal of Psychiatry, 160*, 636–645.

Gruber, B. L., & Taub, E. (1998). Thermal and EMG biofeedback learning in nonhuman primates. *Applied Psychophysiology and Biofeedback, 23*, 1–12.

Gunkelman, J. (2006). Transcend the DSM using phenotypes. *Biofeedback, 34*, 95–98.

Gunkelman, J. (2009). *Drug exposure and EEG/qEEG findings*. qEEEsupport.com.

Gunkelman, J. (2014). Medication prediction with electroencephalography phenotypes and biomarkers. *Biofeedback, 42*(2), 68–73.

Hammond, D. C. (2005). Neurofeedback with anxiety and affective disorders. *Child and Adolescent Psychiatric Clinics of North America, 14*, 105–123.

Hammond, D. C. (2006a). Quantitative electroencephalography patterns associated with medical conditions. *Biofeedback, 34*, 87–94.

Hammond, D. C. (2006b). What is neurotherapy? *Journal of Neurotherapy, 10*, 25–36.

Hanslmayr, S., Sauseng, P., Doppelmayr, M., Schabus, M., & Klimesch, W. (2005). Increasing individual upper alpha power by neurofeedback improves cognitive performance in human subjects. *Applied Psychophysiology and Biofeedback, 30*, 1–10.

Haverman-Nies, A., & De Groot, W. A. (2003). Dietary quality, lifestyle factors and healthy ageing in Europe: The SENECA study. *Age and Ageing, 32*, 427–434.

Hecht, D. (2010). Depression and the hyperactive right-hemisphere. *Neuroscience Research, 68*(2), 77–87.

Henriques, J. B., & Davidson, R. J. (1990). Regional brain electrical asymmetries discriminate between previously depressed and healthy control subjects. *Journal of Abnormal Psychology, 99*, 22–31.

Hoedlmoser, K., Pecherstorfer, T., Gruber, E., Anderer, P., Doppelmayr, M., Klimesch, W., et al. (2008). Instrumental conditioning of human sensorimotor rhythm (12–15 Hz) and its impact on sleep as well as declarative learning. *Sleep, 31*(10), 1401–1408.

Hughes, J. R., & John, E. R. (1999). Conventional and quantitative electroencephalography in psychiatry. *The Journal of Neuropsychiatry and Clinical Neurosciences, 11*, 190–206.

Ingram, R. E. & Luxon, D. D. (2005). Vulnerability-Stress Models. In B. L. Hankin & J. R. Z. Abela (Eds.) *Development of psychopathology: A vulnerability stress perspective* (pp.32–46). Thousand Oaks, CA: Sage.

Itil, T. M., Marasa, J., Saletu, B., Davis, S., & Mucciardi, A. N. (1975). Computerized EEG: Predictor of outcome in schizophrenia. *The Journal of Nervous and Mental Disease, 160*, 118–203.

Jann, K., Koenig, T., Dierks, T., Boesch, C., & Federspiel, A. (2010). Association of individual resting states EEG alpha frequency and cerebral blood flow. *Neuroimaging, 51*(1), 365–372.

Jasper, H., & Shagass, C. (1941). Conditioning the alpha rhythm in man. *Journal of Experimental Psychology, 28*(5), 373–388.

Jin, Y., Potkin, S. G., Kemp, A. S., Huerta, S. T., Alva, G., Thai, T. M., et al. (2006). Therapeutic effects of individualized alpha frequency transcranial magnetic stimulation (alphaTMS) on the negative symptoms of schizophrenia. *Schizophrenia Bulletin, 32*, 556–561.

Johnstone, J. (2005). Clinical database development: Characterization of EEG phentotypes. *Clinical EEG and Neuroscience, 36*, 99–107.

Journal of Abnormal Psychology (2005). Special Section: Toward a Dimensionally Based Taxonomy of Psychopathology. Volume 114(4), pp. 491–569.

Kalogeropoulos, A. P., Georgiopoulou, V. V., & Butler, J. (2012). From risk factors to structural heart disease: The role of inflammation. *Heart Failure Clinics, 8*, 113–123.

Kamiya, J. (1968). Conscious control of brain waves. *Psychology Today, 1*(11), 56–60.

Kang, D., Davidson, R. J., Coe, L. C., Wheeler, R. E., & Tomarken, A. J. (1991). Frontal brain asymmetry and immune function. *Behavioral Neuroscience, 105*(6), 860–869.

Kanoh, S., Murayama, Y. M., Miyamoto, K., Yoshinobu, T., & Kawashima, R. (2009). A NIRS-based brain-computer interface system during motor imagery: System development and online feedback training. In *Conference Proceedings: Annual International Conference of the IEEE Engineering in Medicine and Biology Society. IEEE Engineering in Medicine and Biology Society Conference, 2009* (pp. 594–597).

Katzmarzyk, P. T. & Lee, I. M. (2012) Sedentary behaviour and life expectancy in the USA: a cause-deleted life table analysis. *BMJ Open 2012;2:e000828* doi:10.1136/bmjopen-2012-000828.

Kessler, R., Adler, L., Barkley, R., Biederman, J., Conners, C., Demler, O., et al. (2006). The prevalence and correlates of adult ADHD in the United States: Results from the National Comorbidity Survey replication. *American Journal of Psychiatry, 163*, 716–723.

Kim, C. H., Chang, J. W., Koo, J. W., Suh, H. S., Park, I. H., & Lee, H. S. (2003). Anterior cingulotomy for refractory obsessive-compulsive disorder. *Acta Psychiatrica Scandinavica, 107*(4), 283–290.

Klimesch, W. (1999). EEG alpha and theta oscillations reflect cognitive and memory performance: A review and analysis. *Brain Research Reviews, 29*, 169–195.

Klimesch, W., Schimke, H., Ladurner, G., & Pfurtscheller, G. (1990a). Alpha frequency and memory performance. *Journal of Psychophysiology, 4*, 381–390.

Klimesch, W., Schimke, H., & Pfurtscheller, G. (1990b). The topography of alpha frequency and memory performance. *Journal of Psychophysiology, 4*, 4191–4192.

Klimesch, W., Schimke, H., & Pfurtscheller, G. (1993). Alpha frequency, cognitive load and memory performance. *Brain Topography, 5*(3), 241–251.

Koberda, J. L., Hillies, D. S., Jones, B., Moses, A., & Koberda, L. (2012). Application of neurofeedback in general neurology practice. *Journal of Neurotherapy, 16*(3), 231–234.

Kostyunina, M. B. (1998). Human EEG during mental reproduction of emotionally significant events. *Zhurnal Vysshei Nervnoi Deyatel'nosti Imeni I P Pavlova, 48*(2), 213–221.

Kostyunina, M. B., & Kulikov, M. A. (1995). Frequency characteristics of different emotions: EEG spectral analysis. *Zhurnal Vysshei Nervnoi Deyatel'nosti Imeni I P Pavlova, 45*(3), 453–457.

Kuczenski, R., & Segal, D. S. (1997). Effects of methylphenidate on extracellular dopamine, serotonin, and norepinephrine: Comparison with amphetamine. *Journal of Neurochemistry, 68*, 2032–2037.

Lander, E. S. (2011). Initial impact of the sequencing of the human genome. *Nature, 470*, 187–197.

Larsen, S. (2006). *The healing power of neurofeedback*. Rochester, VT: Healing Arts Press.

LeDoux, J. (2002). *Synaptic self: How our brains become who we are*. New York, Viking.

Lehrer, P. (2013). How does heart rate variability biofeedback work? Resonance, the baroreflex, and other mechanisms. *Biofeedback, 41*, 26–31.

Lennox-Buchal, M., Buchtal, F., & Rosenfalck, P. (1960). Correlation of electroencephalographic findings with crash rate of military jet pilots. *Epilepsia, 1*, 366–372.

Lipton, B. (2006) Biology of Belief. Carlsbad, CA: Hay House

Lubar, J. F. (1991). Discourse on the development of EEG diagnostics and biofeedback treatment for attention-deficit/hyperactivity disorders. *Biofeedback and Self-Regulation, 16*, 201–225.

Lubar, J. F., & Bahler, W. W. (1976). Behavioral management of epileptic seizures following biofeedback training of the sensorimotor rhythm. *Biofeedback and Self-Regulation, 1*, 77–104.

Lubar, J. F., & Shouse, M. N. (1977). Use of biofeedback in the treatment of seizure disorders and hyperactivity. *Advances in Clinical Child Psychology, 1*, 204–251.

Luby, J. L., Gaffrey, M. S., Tillman, R., April, L. M., & Belden, A. C. (2014). Trajectories of preschool disorders to full DSM depression at school age and early adolescence: Continuity of preschool depression. *American Journal of Psychiatry, 171*, 768–776.

Maurage, P., Campanella, S., Philippot, P., Vermeulen, N., Constant, E., Luminet, O., et al. (2008). Electrophysiological correlates of the disrupted processing of anger in alcoholism. *International Journal of Psychophysiology, 70*(1), 50–62.

Miller, V., Mocroft, A., Reiss, P., Kaglama, C., Papadopoulos, A. I., Katzenstein, T., et al. (1999). Relations among CD4 lymphocyte count nadir, antiretroviral therapy, and HIV-1 disease progression. *Annals of Internal Medicine, 130*, 570–577.

Monastra, V. J., Monastra, D. M., & Geogre, S. (2002). The effects of stimulant therapy, EEG biofeedback and parenting style on the primary symptoms of attention-deficit/hyperactivity disorder. *Journal of Applied Psychophysiology and Biofeedback, 27*, 231–249.

National Scientific Council on the Developing Child. (2005). *Excessive stress disrupts the architecture of the developing brain* (Working Paper No. 3). www.developingchild.harvard.edu.

Ng, S. C., & Raveendran, P. (2007). EEG peak alpha frequency as an indicator of physical fatigue. In T. Jarm, P. Kramar, & A. Zupanic (Eds.), *Medicon 2007, IFMBE Proceedings 16* (pp. 517–520).

Nüesch, E., Häuser, W., Bernardy, K., Barth, J., & Jüni, P. (2013). Comparative efficacy of pharmacological and non-pharmacological interventions in fibromyalgia syndrome: Network meta-analysis. *Annals of the Rheumatic Diseases, 72*, 955–962.

Oatley, K., Keltner, D., & Jenkins, J. M. (2006). *Emotions and mental health in childhood. Understanding emotions* (2nd ed., pp. 321–351). Oxford, UK: Blackwell Publishing.

Odden, M. C., Peralta, C. A., Haan, M. N., & Covinsky, K. E. (2012). Rethinking the association of high blood pressure with mortality in elderly adults: The impact of frailty. *Archives of Internal Medicine, 172*(15), 1162–1168.

Ohatrian, G. E., Peterson, M. C., & Lazarre, J. A. (1960). Responses from clicks from the human brain: Some depth electrographic observations. *Electroencephalography and Clinical Neurophysiology, 12*, 479–489.

Ohayon, M. M., Reynolds, C. F., 3rd, & Dauvilliers, Y. (2013). Excessive sleep duration and quality of life. *Annals of Neurology, 73*(6), 785–794.

Okamura, H., Jing, H., & Takigawa, M. (2001). EEG modification induced by repetitive transcranial magnetic stimulation. *Journal of Clinical Neurophysiology, 18*, 318–325.

Olding, S. (2008). *Pathologies*. Calgary, AB: Freehand Press.

Osaka, M. (1984). Peak alpha frequency of EEG during a mental task: Task difficulty and hemispheric differences. *Psychophysiology, 21*(1), 101–105.

Oudiette, D., Antony, J. W., Creery, J. C., & Paller, K. A. (2013). The role of memory reactivation during wakefulness and sleep in determining which memories endure. *Journal of Neuroscience, 33*, 6672–6678.

Parmeggiani, A., Barcia, G., Posar, A., Raimondi, E., Santucci, M., & Scaduto, M. C. (2010). Epilepsy EEG paroxysmal abnormalities in autism spectrum disorders. *Brain and Development, 32*, 783–789.

Peniston, E. G., & Kulkosky, P. J. (1999). Neurofeedback in the treatment of addictive disorders. In J. R. Evans & A. Abarbanel (Eds.), *Introduction to quantitative EEG and neurofeedback* (pp. 157–179). New York: Academic Press.

Pfurtscheller, G., Steffan, J., & Maresch, H. (1988). ERD mapping and functional topography: Temporal and spatial aspects. In G. Pfurtscheller & F. H. Lopez da Silva (Eds.), *Functional brain imaging* (pp. 117–130). Toronto: Hans Huber.

Piacentini, J. (2014). 24- and 36-week outcomes for the Child/Adolescent Anxiety Multimodal Study (CAMS). *Journal of the American Academy of Child and Adolescent Psychiatry, 53*(3), 297–310.

Pittman, S. D., MacDonald, M. M., Fogel, R. B., Malhotra, A.,Todros, K., Levy, B., et al. (2004). Assessment of automated scoring of polysomnographic recordings in a population with suspected sleep-disordered breathing. *Sleep, 27*(7), 1394–1403.

Porjesz, B., Almasy, L., Edenberg, H., Wang, K., Chorlian, D. B., Foroud, T., et al. (2002). Linkage disequilibrium between the beta frequency of the human EEG and a GABAA receptor gene locus. *Proceedings of the National Academy of Sciences of the United States of America, 99*, 3729–3733.

Prinloo, G. E., Rauch, H. G., Karpul, D., & Derman, W. E. (2013). The effect of a single session of short duration heart rate variability biofeedback on EEG: A pilot study. *Applied Psychophysiology and Biofeedback, 38*, 45–56.

Rangaswamy, M., Porjesz, B., Chorlian, D. B., Wang, K., Jones, K. A., Bauer, L. O., et al. (2002). Beta power in the EEG of alcoholics. *Biological Psychiatry, 52*, 831–842.

Reeves, R., Struve, F., Patrick, G., & Bullen, J. (1995). Topographic quantitative EEG measures of alpha and theta power changes during caffeine withdrawal: Preliminary findings from normal subjects. *Clinical EEG and Neuroscience, 26*, 154–162.

Reid, A., & Nihon, S. (2011). *Effects of heart rate variability training on sensory motor rhythm amplitude*. Presentation at the ISNR annual conference, Phoenix, AZ.

Reid, A., Nihon, S., Thompson, L., & Thompson, M. (2013). The effects of heart rate variability training on sensorimotor rhythm: A pilot study. *Journal of Neurotherapy, 17*, 43–48.

Ritchlin, C. T., Chabot, R. J., Alper, K., Buyon, J., Belmont, H. M., Roubey, R., et al. (1992). Quantitative electroencephalography: A new approach to the diagnosis of cerebral dysfunction in systemic lupus erythematosus. *Arthritis and Rheumatism, 35*, 1330–1342.

Rizzuto, D., Orsini, N., Qiu, C., Wang, H.-X., & Fratiglioni, L. (2012). Lifestyle, social factors, and survival after age 75: Population based study. *British Medical Journal, 10*, 1136.

Robbins, J. (2000). *A symphony in the brain*. New York: Grove Press. An interesting account of Sterman's work can be found in this reference.
Rösler, M., Retz, W., Retz-Junginger, P., Hengesch, G., Schneider, M., Supprian, T., et al. (2004). Prevalence of Attention Deficit/Hyperactivity Disorder (ADHD) and comorbid disorders in young male prison inmates. *European Archives of Psychiatry and Clinical Neuroscience, 254*, 365–371.
Roth, M., Kay, D. W., Shaw, J., & Green, J. (1957). Prognosis and pentothal induced electroencephalographic changes in electroconvulsive treatment; an approach to the problem of regulation of convulsive therapy. *Electroencephalography and Clinical Neurophysiology, 9*, 225–237.
Sakusic, A., Avdibegovic, E., Zoricic, Z., Pavlovic, S., Gaspar, V., & Delic, A. (2010). Relationship between anger, alcoholism and symptoms of posttraumatic stress disorders in war veterans. *Medicinski Arhiv, 64*(6), 354–358.
Salinsky, M., Binder, L., Oken, B., Storzbach, D., Aron, C., & Dodrill, C. (2002). Effects of gabapentin and carbamazepine on the EEG and cognition in healthy volunteers. *Epilepsia, 43*, 482–490.
Salinsky, M., Oken, B., & Morehead, L. (1994). Intra-individual analysis of antiepileptic drug effects on EEG background rhythms. *Electroencephalography and Clinical Neurophysiology, 90*, 186–193.
Schwartz, M. S., & Andrasik, F. (2005). *Biofeedback: A practitioner's guide* (3rd ed.). New York, NY: Guilford Press.
Schwartz, R. B., Komaroff, A. L., Garada, B. M., Gleit, M., Doolittle, T. H., Bates, D. W., et al. (1994). SPECT imaging of the brain: Comparison of findings in patients with chronic fatigue syndrome, AIDS dementia complex, and major unipolar depression. *American Journal of Roentgenology, 162*, 943–951.
Seifer, R., Dickstein, S., Sameroff, A. J., Magee, K. D., & Hayden, L. C. (2001). Infant mental health and variability of parental depression symptoms. *Journal of the American Academy of Child and Adolescent Psychiatry, 40*, 1375–1382.
Shambroom, J. R., Fabregas, S. E., & Johnstone, J. (2011). Validation of an automated wireless system to monitor sleep in healthy adults. *Journal of Sleep Research, 21*, 221–230.
Shummer, G. J., Noh, S. M., & Mendoza, J. J. (2013). The effect of neurofeedback and cranial electrotherapy on immune function within a group of HIV+ subjects: A controlled study. *Journal of Neurotherapy, 17*, 151–161.
Sigelman, C.K. & Rider, E.A. (2009). *Developmental psychopathology. Life-span human development* (6th ed., pp. 468–495). Belmont, CA: Wadsworth Cengage Learning.
Simon, G., & Perlis, R. H. (2010). Personalized medicine for depression: Can we match patients with treatments? *American Journal of Psychiatry, 16*, 1445–1455.
Sterman, M. B. (2000). An interesting account of Sterman's work can be found in Jim Robbins (2000). *A symphony in the brain*. New York: Grove Press.
Stephens, J. R., Heffner, J. L., Adler, C. A., Blom, T. J., Anthenelli, R. M., Fleck, D. E., et al. (2014). Risk and protective factors associated with substance use disorders in adolescents with first-episode mania. *Journal of the American Academy of Child and Adolescent Psychiatry, 53*, 771–779.
Sterman, M. B., & Egner, T. (2006). Foundation and practice of neurofeedback for the treatment of epilepsy. *Applied Psychophysiology and Biofeedback, 31*(1), 21–36.
Suffin, S. C., & Emory, W. H. (1995). Neurometric subgroups in attentional and affective disorders and their association with pharmacotherapeutic outcome. *Clinical Electroencephalography, 26*(2), 76–83.
Swingle, P. G. (1992, August). *Subliminal treatment procedures*. In Symposium entitled "Subliminal influences: For better or for naught?", American Psychological Association Meeting, Washington, DC.
Swingle, P. G. (1992a). *Subliminal treatment procedures: A clinician's guide*. Sarasota, FL: Professional Resource Press.

Swingle, P. G. (1993, June). *Subliminal facilitation.* Invited Workshop. International Conference on Transcultural Psychiatry, Montreal, Quebec.

Swingle, P. G. (1994). Clinical applications of subliminal auditory stimulation: The treatment of attention deficiency. In R. Kall, J. Kamiya, & G. Swartz (Eds.), *Applied psychophysiology and brainwave biofeedback.* Newtown, PA: Futurehealth.

Swingle, P. G. (1995, February). *Somatosensory effects on brainwave architecture in neuronal therapy.* Paper presented at the Futurehealth Conference, Advances in Neurotherapy, Key West, FL.

Swingle, P. G. (1996). Subthreshold 10 Hz sound suppresses EEG Theta: Clinical application for the potentiation of neurotherapy treatment of ADD/ADHD. *Journal of Neurotherapy, 2*(1), 15–22.

Swingle, P. G. (1997, February). *Artifact problems in EEG biofeedback.* Paper presented at the Futurehealth Conference, Advances in Neurotherapy, Palm Springs, CA.

Swingle, P.G. (1998, February) *Adjunctive treatment procedures.* Paper presented at the Futurehealth Conference Advances in Neurotherapy. Palm Springs, CA.

Swingle, P. G. (1998a). Neurofeedback treatment of pseudoseizure disorder. *Biological Psychiatry, 44*, 1196–1199.

Swingle, P. G. (1998, February). *Adjunctive treatment procedures.* Paper presented at the Futurehealth Conference, Advances in Neurotherapy, Palm Springs, CA.

Swingle, P. G. (2001). Parameters associated with the rapid neurotherapeutic treatment of Common ADD (CADD). *Journal of Neurotherapy, 5*(4), 73–84.

Swingle, P. G. (2002, February). *Clinical applications of the QuickQ diagnostic brain assessment.* Paper presented at the Futurehealth Winterbrain Conference, Palm Springs, CA.

Swingle, P. G. (2003, February). *Emotional release techniques facilitate enhancement of occipital theta amplitude in patients with severe traumatic stress.* Paper presented at the Futurehealth Winterbrain Conference, Palm Springs, CA.

Swingle, P. G. (2003, Summer). Potentiating neurotherapy: Techniques for stimulating the EEG. *California Biofeedback.*

Swingle, P. G. (2006, April). *Assessment and treatment of emotional trauma.* Paper presented at the Association of Applied Psychophysiology and Biofeedback Meeting, Portland, OR.

Swingle, P.G. (2008) *Biofeedback for the Brain.* New Brunswick, N.J., Rutgers University Press.

Swingle, P. G. (2010). *Biofeedback for the brain.* New Brunswick, NJ: Rutgers University Press.

Swingle, P. G. (2013). The effects of negative emotional stimuli on alpha blunting. *Journal of Neurotherapy, 17*(2), 133–138.

Tansey, M. A. (1986). A simple and a complex tic (Gilles de la Tourette's syndrome): Their response to EEG sensorimotor rhythm biofeedback training. *International Journal of Psychophysiology, 4*(2), 91–97.

Thompson, M., Nihon, S., Thompson, L., & Thompson, M. (2013). The effects of heart rate variability training on sensorimotor rhythm: A pilot study. *Journal of Neurotherapy, 17*, 43–48.

Thompson, M., & Thompson, L. (2006). Improving attention in adults and children: Differing electroencephalographic profiles and implications for training. *Biofeedback, 34*, 99–105.

Thompson, M., & Thompson, L. (2011, Winter). Improving quality of life using biofeedback plus neurofeedback. *Neuroconnections*, 18–21

Thornton, K. (2006). Subtype analysis of learning disability by quantitative electroencephalography patterns. *Biofeedback, 34*, 106–113.

Tinius, T. (Ed.). (2004). *New developments in blood flow hemoencephalography.* Binghamton, NY: Haworth Medical Press.

Toomim, H., Mize, W., Kwong, P. C., Toomim, M., Marsh, R., Kozlowski, G. P., et al. (2004). Intentional increase of cerebral blood oxygenation using hemoencephalography (HEG): An efficient brain exercise therapy. *Journal of Neurotherapy, 8*, 5–21.

Torres, F., Faoro, R., Lowenson, R., & Johnson, E. (1983). The electroencephalogram of elderly subjects revisited. *Electroencephalography and Clinical Neurophysiology, 66*, 391–398.

Tronick, E., & Reck, C. (2009). Infants of depressed mothers. *Harvard Review of Psychiatry, 17*, 147–156.
Ulrich, G., Renfordt, E., Zeller, G., & Frick, K. (1984). Interrelation between changes in the EEG and psychopathology under pharmacotherapy for endogenous depression. *A contribution to the predictor question. Pharmacopsychiatry, 17*, 178–183.
van Beijsterveldt, C. E. (2002). Twin and family studies of the human electroencephalogram: A review and a meta-analysis. *Biological Psychology, 61*, 111–138.
van Lieshout, E. J., van der Veer, S. N., Hensbroek, R., Korevaar, J. C., Vroom, M. B., & Schultz, M. J. (2007). Interference by new-generation mobile phones on critical care medical equipment. *Critical Care, 11*(5), R98.
Vieta, E., Thase, M. E., Naber, D., et al. (2014). Efficacy and tolerability of flexibly-dosed adjunct TC-5214 (dexmecamylamine) in patients with major depressive disorder and inadequate response to prior antidepressants. *European Neuropsychopharmacology, 24*, 564–574.
Wahbeh, H., & Oken, B. S. (2013). Peak high-frequency HRV and peak alpha frequency higher in PTSD. *Applied Psychophysiology and Biofeedback, 38*, 57–69.
Westmoreland, B. F. (1993). The EEG in cerebral inflammatory processes. In E. E. Neidermyer & F. L. DaSilva (Eds.), *Electroencephalography: Basic principles, clinical applications and related fields* (3rd ed., pp. 291–304). Philadelphia: Lippincott Williams & Wilkins.
Wolters, E. C., van der Werf, Y. D., & van den Heuvel, O. A. (2008). Parkinson's disease-related disorders in the impulsive-compulsive spectrum". *Journal of Neurology, 255*(Suppl. 5), 48–56.
Yasuhara, A. (2010) Correlation between EEG abnormalities and symptoms of autism spectrum disorder (ASD). *Brain Development, 32*(10), 791–798.
Young, S., Toone, B., & Tyson, C. (2002). Comorbidity and psychosocial profile of adults with Attention Deficit Hyperactivity Disorder. *Personality and Individual Differences, 35*, 743–755.
Yutaka, I., Teicher, M. H., Glod, R. N., & Ackerman, B. S. (1998). Preliminary evidence for aberrant cortical development in abused children. *Journal of Neuropsychiatry and Clinical Neurosciences, 10*, 298–307.
Zoefel, B., Huster, R. J., & Herrmann, C. S. (2011). Neurofeedback training of the upper alpha frequency band in EEG improves cognitive performance. *Journal of Neuroimaging, 54*(2), 1427–1431.

Index

P.G. Swingle, *Adding Neurotherapy to Your Practice*,
DOI 10.1007/978-3-319-15527-2

Lightning Source UK Ltd.
Milton Keynes UK
UKHW021315161222
414044UK00001B/1

9 783319 155265